beating
back pain

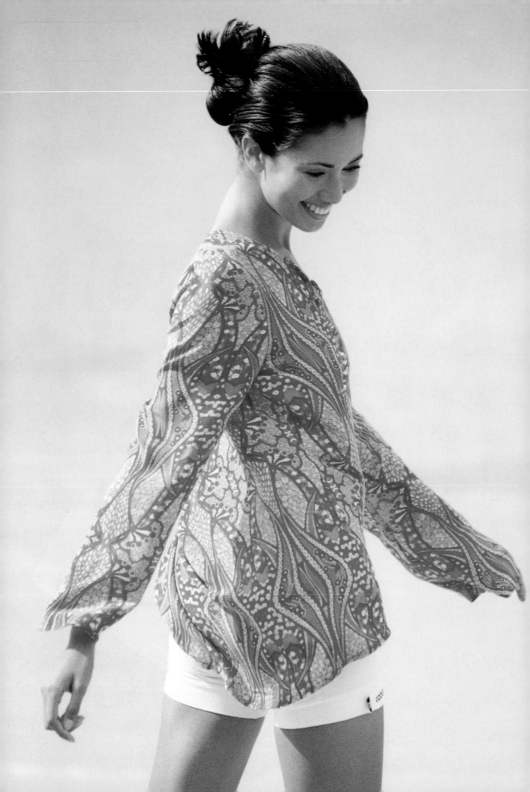

beating
back pain

through conventional and alternative methods

anthony campbell
MRCP (U.K.), Dip. Med. Ac., FF. Hom

Consultants
Dr. Len Saputo
Dr. Richard Gracer

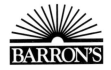

First edition for the United States, its territories and dependencies, and Canada published in 2003 by Barron's Educational Series, Inc.

First published in Great Britain in 2003 by Mitchell Beazley, under the title *Options for Health: Beating Back Pain*.

Mitchell Beazley is an imprint of Octopus Publishing Group Ltd, 2-4 Heron Quays, Docklands, London E14 4JP

All inquiries should be addressed to:
Barron's Educational Series, Inc.
250 Wireless Boulevard
Hauppauge, NY 11788
http://www.barronseduc.com

International Standard Book No.: 0-7641-2040-9

Library of Congress Catalog Card No.: 2003102211

Executive Editor	Vivien Antwi
Executive Art Editor	Christine Keilty
Project Editor	Naomi Waters
Design	Alexa Brommer
Copy Editors	Rona Johnson and Adrian Morgan
Picture Research	Emma O'Neill
Proofreader	Siobhan O' Connor
Indexer	Sandra Shotter
Production	Alexis Coogan
Medical Consultants	Len Saputo and Richard Gracer

Picture Credits
Front cover BananaStock; 2 Getty Images/V.C.L; 12 Getty Images/Ghislaine & Marie David de Lossy; 15 & 16 Science Photo Library/John Bavosi; 18 Corbis/Pete Saloutos; 19 Robert Harding Picture Library/Siri Mills/Phototake NYC; 21 Science Photo Library; 25 Corbis/Jon Feingersh; 29 Science Photo Library/GJLP; 33 Corbis/Mauro Panci; 38 Science Photo Library/John Bavosi; 40 Robert Harding Picture Library/GJLP./CNRI/Phototake NYC; 45 & 52 ImageState; 55 Corbis/Michael Keller; 56 Corbis/LWA-JDC; 59 Corbis; 61 ImageState; 63 Octopus Publishing Group/Niki Sianni; 65 Getty Images/Gary Buss; 67 Corbis/Ariel Skelley; 70 Getty Images/Jean-Marc Scialom; 74 Octopus Publishing Group/Simon Smith; 79 BananaStock; 80 Getty Images/Mark Williams; 82 Robert Harding Picture Library/Art Brewer/Int'l Stock; 95 Corbis/Tom & Dee Ann McCarthy; 96 Getty Images/Robert Daly; 98 Getty Images/Deborah Jaffe; 103 Corbis/Norbert Schaefer; 106 Corbis/Pete Saloutos; 109 Photodisc; 111 Corbis; 115 Corbis/Charles Gupton; 117, 118, 123, 124 & 127 Corbis; 130 Photodisc; 134 Octopus Publishing Group/Mark Winwood

Publisher's note: Before following any advice or exercises contained in this book, it is recommended that you consult your doctor if you suffer from any health problems or special conditions. The publishers cannot accept responsibility for any injuries or damage incurred as a result of following the advice given in this book.

Typeset in Futura and Folio

Printed and bound by Toppan Printing Company, China
9 8 7 6 5 4 3 2 1

contents

foreword

If you suffer from back pain there is hope – there is an effective treatment plan for nearly everyone. There are more options to treat back pain today than there have ever been before. Our modern treatments combine the most sophisticated technology with time-tested healing systems, as well as cutting-edge alternatives. In fact, there are so many options that it takes an expert in both conventional and alternative medicine to sort through which therapies are most appropriate for each individual person. This is one of the main reasons *Beating Back Pain* was written.

As he wrote this book, Anthony Campbell collected and organized an enormous amount of literature in a form that is highly informative and easily readable. It will help readers to make informed decisions about how to get started in beating their back pain, and empower them to take a more active role in making wise healthcare choices. After all, it is important to understand the therapies recommended by our healthcare practitioners. We are the ones who will live with the consequences.

Dr. Campbell begins with an overview describing the basic anatomy of the back, what symptoms are typically associated with specific back problems, and how you can determine what is wrong if you have back symptoms. He reviews a wide variety of conditions such as injuries, neck and lower-back disk problems, osteoporosis, and even the backache of pregnancy.

Most back problems are preventable. Usually, they do not need to develop. Taking care of your back by eating a nutritious diet, enjoying proper exercise, getting adequate sleep, and adopting a good mental outlook – having a healthy lifestyle – can make the difference between having a strong back and suffering from an unnecessary disability. Advice on how to adapt these approaches to your particular lifestyle and to your particular back problem will help you develop routines that are proactive in restoring and maintaining a healthy back. You will also learn when it is important to see your medical doctor.

There is a tremendous range of possible approaches that can be used in managing the pain of both acute and chronic back conditions. In this book, treatment options are reviewed from the perspective of many disciplines, and approaches are offered that will appeal to most patients. It is important to remember that it is possible, and often beneficial, to combine therapies. Collaboration can synergize outcomes that speed recovery times, result in highly cost-effective strategies, offer more options that provide greater safety, and involve patients more directly in making their own healthcare choices. Because we are all different, our needs and preferences vary, and the treatment programs we choose should be individualized accordingly.

Dr. Campbell looks beyond the physical dimension, paying attention to the whole person – body, mind, and spirit – as he considers options for treatment. By addressing the emotional aspects of pain and disability through therapy, imagery, and psychological counseling, better outcomes are achieved more often. The importance of posttraumatic stress syndrome in people with prolonged disabilities, especially those resulting from injuries or who have had multiple surgeries, is now widely appreciated by modern medicine. This syndrome is far more common than previously believed, and is now typically treated by teams of practitioners that often include primary care physicians, physical therapists, and psychologists.

Included in this book is an explanation of how different disciplines such as mainstream medicine, osteopathy, homeopathy, herbal medicine, chiropractic, acupuncture, nutrition, psychology, and various types of exercise and physical therapy can contribute to assessing and managing back pain. The strengths and weaknesses of these styles of healthcare are highlighted, making it practical for you to consider which ones are appropriate for your specific needs. In addition, new high-tech therapies such as infrared light therapy (photonic stimulation), that are on the horizon and hold promise as powerful adjuncts to what is possible to relieve pain and promote healing, are presented.

So, yes, there is hope for everyone who has back pain. You are most likely to get the best possible results by working in collaboration with your healthcare practitioner. As you read this book, you will appreciate that it is realistic to take an active role in managing your own healthcare choices. There are a wide variety of approaches that can fit your uniquely individual needs, and they are not beyond your comprehension.

Len Saputo, M.D.

introduction

Back pain can take many forms. A young person may suffer a "stiff neck" on waking one morning; it comes on suddenly, for no apparent reason, and disappears as mysteriously after a few days. A middle-aged man digs in his garden one Sunday in the spring and wakes up next morning to find his lower back stiff and painful, recognizing what has happened because he has suffered from "lumbago" previously. A woman loads shopping into her car, twisting her back awkwardly as she does so, and that evening experiences a dull ache in the lower part of her back, which persists all the following day. On the second morning she wakes to find that her back is so stiff that she cannot put on her shoes and she is in constant severe pain. Later the pain eases somewhat in her back but instead she begins to experience severe pain in her leg – sciatica. A fit young man bends forward to pick something up from the ground and suddenly his back "locks" so that he cannot move or straighten himself.

These are just some of the ways in which back pain may occur. But in spite of the importance of the problem, it can be surprisingly difficult to get firm answers to the question of why it happens. We are sometimes told that it is due to our "unnatural" upright stance; if we walked on all fours, the argument runs, we would not suffer from back problems. But in fact, quadrupeds do suffer in this way, and our species or its forerunners have walked upright for over a million years so it seems unlikely that we have failed to adapt to it by now.

For whatever reasons, however, back pain is common in our western society. Probably you, or someone you know, has experienced it. In 1993, 11 percent of the British population reported that their activities had been restricted by back pain in the last four weeks. In the United States the estimated annual cost to society of back pain is between $20 billion and $50 billion; back symptoms are the most common cause of disability in people under 45; about half of all working adults report a back injury each year, and about one percent of the population is chronically disabled by back pain. Figures for other industrialized countries are similar. In Britain there was a five-fold increase in outpatient treatments for back pain in the decade to 1993, and the number of days for which disability benefits were paid more than doubled.

This may sound alarming, but it is important to keep a sense of proportion about it. The media sometimes talks about an "epidemic" of back pain but the evidence for such a thing is really not very good. It is likely that much of the apparent increase in back pain is explained by cultural changes, which make people more aware of minor back symptoms and more willing to seek help for them. Back pain is now more acceptable as a reason for absence from work. Two surveys in Britain, conducted 10 years apart, indicate that while there has been no increase in the incidence of severe, disabling back pain, the incidence of less disabling back pain has increased, which again suggests that cultural factors are important.

There are 8.5 million GP consultations in Britain for back pain every year, but only about 25,000 people make the transition from short-term to long-term disability payments. The good news, therefore, is that if you suffer an episode of acute back pain the chances that you will progress to chronic disability are very small. Most people get better. It also suggests that acute and chronic back pain are different from the outset; chronic back pain is not just acute pain that goes on longer.

This book looks at what is currently known about back pain: its causes, prevention, and treatment. Our knowledge about these things is constantly increasing and new ideas are emerging all the time. There have been three main areas of change in our thinking. First, it is now recognized that pain, and especially long-lasting pain, is much more complicated than was understood previously. This has led to new ways of coping with pain, in which multiple approaches are used simultaneously — both more effective and more realistic in terms of what can and cannot be achieved in pain of this kind.

Second, there has been a change in attitudes to so-called alternative medicine. A few decades ago treatments such as osteopathy, chiropractic, and acupuncture were regarded by most doctors as useless or even potentially harmful. Today, many doctors, along with other health professionals, are either using these forms of treatment themselves or are at least willing to refer their patients to people who practice them. This is particularly true in the case of back pain. The boundaries between mainstream and alternative therapies are becoming blurred: for example, physiotherapists often use manipulative treatments that originated with the osteopaths. Another sign of this change in attitude has been the quite frequent appearance of research articles on unorthodox therapies in leading mainstream medical journals.

The third development underlies both conventional and alternative treatments for back pain. This is the request for evidence of effectiveness. In all the developed countries demands on health services have increased very greatly, but resources are limited, so not everything can be afforded. It is therefore considered essential for the effectiveness of the treatments offered to have been demonstrated objectively. This has led to a great increase in the number of clinical trials being carried out. So many are being done, in fact, that it is all but impossible for most therapists to keep abreast of the information; hence the need for critical reviews of the research. This matters not only to the governments who have to fund their health services, but also it matters to us as individuals. If you have back pain you want to know which treatments are likely to help; you also want to know if they can do harm. Although it is true that full information about the effectiveness of many treatments is not yet available, so that we may often have to proceed on a balance of probabilities rather than absolute certainty, it still makes sense to be aware of what knowledge does exist.

Fortunately, objective information of this kind is now becoming increasingly available both to health professionals and to their patients. Many people nowadays turn to the Internet, which provides so much material that it is difficult to find one's way through it; but a few sites stand out above the rest. Among these, perhaps the most useful is the Cochrane Library, published electronically by the Cochrane Collaboration and available to the general public in many countries including Britain and the United States. This international organization publishes high-quality evidence to inform people providing and receiving care. In order to ensure that this book is as up to date as possible, much of the advice and recommendations here are based on Cochrane Library material.

The book is divided into two main parts, Understanding Back Pain and Options for a Healthy Back, each of which is subdivided into chapters. The first chapter within Understanding Back Pain describes the structure and function of the back. It is essential to have a mental picture of this in order to understand the descriptions of what can go wrong. If the information is new to you, it is not essential to take it all in at once. You may prefer to move on through the book and refer back to the first section in order to clarify particular questions. The glossary also provides a quick summary of the important concepts and relevant medical terms.

The next chapter is about what can go wrong with the back and describes the symptoms and causes of all the common problems as well as a few of the more unusual ones. The next chapter covers methods of diagnosis.

Part Two, Options for a Healthy Back, opens with a range of preventive measures that you can build in to your daily life in order to reduce your risk of back pain. The second chapter explains why exercising to promote good general health is also good for your back, but that the value of specific back exercises remains open to debate.

If you suffer from back pain, naturally you want to know what to do about it. In subsequent chapters we therefore look at treatment, which differs according to whether your pain is a first attack or is long-term. Chronic or long-term pain is much the more difficult to deal with and there are various possible approaches, some are conventional, such as surgery, while others, such as manipulation or acupuncture, are generally classed as complementary. As we shall see, however, the gap that is used to separate conventional and complementary treatments is beginning to close. Yet another important development in many centers is the introduction of what is called multidisciplinary rehabilitation, which seeks to make people with long-term back pain better able to function and return to work.

How the tabs work

In the chapters on The Structure of the Back, Symptoms and Their Causes, and Diagnosis in Part One, Understanding Back Pain, are a series of colored tabs. These guide you to the most appropriate therapies, treatments, or preventive measures that are most likely to be useful for treating a particular condition or problem, and relate to the color-coded chapters in Part Two, Options for a Healthy Back. Here you will find more information on these therapies.

Prevention

Exercise

Treatment (Acute)

Treatment (Chronic)

Therapists

Physical Therapies

Natural Therapies

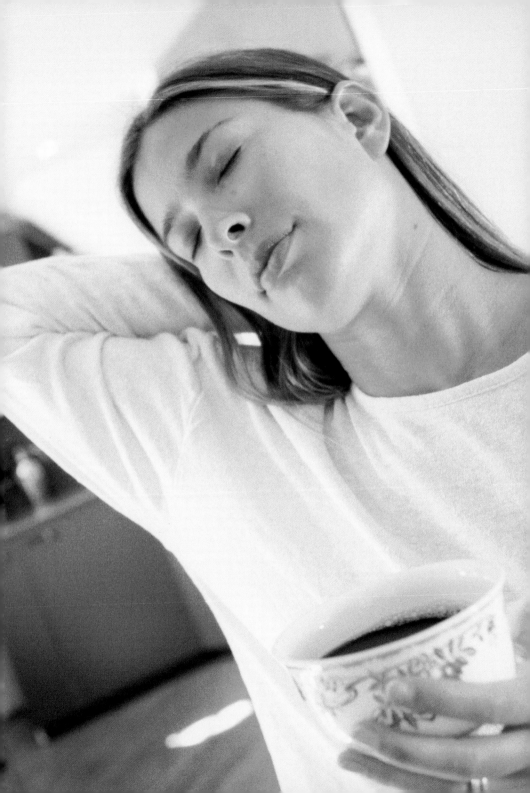

understanding
back
pain

To understand back pain we need to know how the back works. Although it is convenient to discuss its various regions and components separately, they do of course interact with one another. Even as simple an action as picking up a book or turning our head will require the integrated activity of muscles in many parts of our back. This integration is largely performed by a part of the brain called the *cerebellum*, and it depends critically on feedback from the special sensory nerves in the muscles and joints. The inner ear and eyes also have important roles to play. The ears detect movement and acceleration; the eyes are often the first body part to actually move, after which the rest of the nervous system follows. This first half of the book describes the anatomy of the back, pain and other symptoms, illnesses, and diagnoses.

the
structure
of the back

The back is a complex structure, made up of many components. At its core is the spine, on which the stability of the back depends. Many, though not all, of the problems that we experience in our backs, are due to disorders of the spine.

The back consists of a scaffolding of bones, joints, and ligaments, surrounded by muscles that serve both to move the spine and to support it and give it integrity. There are also numerous blood vessels and nerves, and connective tissue that sheathes these structures in a network of fibers. If all the bones and muscles in the body were taken away, the connective tissue background would still be there, like a kind of ghostly outline, to indicate its shape and give the body its ultimate integrity; it stores energy as it stretches and maintains relationships between body parts. It is this tissue, along with the ligaments, that defines shape and function.

The Spine

The spine comprises a column of 26 bones, the vertebrae (sing. vertebra), stacked on top of one another like a pile of coins. It has three major divisions: cervical, thoracic, and lumbar. At the top is the cervical or neck region, made up of seven vertebrae. Below this is the thoracic or chest region, with 12 vertebrae, each of which has a pair of ribs attached to it. The ribs move a fair amount to permit the chest to expand in breathing. Therefore, the rib and vertebral joints are extremely important to spinal function. Problems with these are a significant cause of thoracic pain. Next there is the lumbar or lower back region, with five vertebrae.

THE STRUCTURE OF THE SPINE

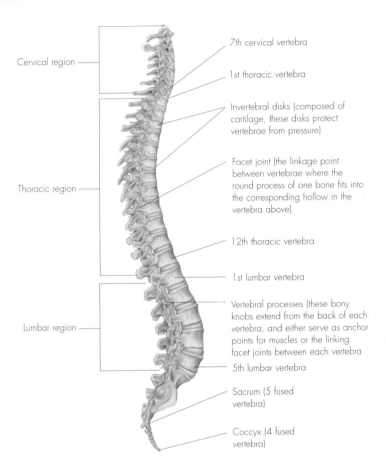

Cervical region

7th cervical vertebra

1st thoracic vertebra

Invertebral disks (composed of cartilage, these disks protect vertebrae from pressure)

Facet joint (the linkage point between vertebrae where the round process of one bone fits into the corresponding hollow in the vertebra above)

Thoracic region

12th thoracic vertebra

1st lumbar vertebra

Vertebral processes (these bony knobs extend from the back of each vertebra, and either serve as anchor points for muscles or the linking facet joints between each vertebra

Lumbar region

5th lumbar vertebra

Sacrum (5 fused vertebra)

Coccyx (4 fused vertebra)

The normal spine: note the gentle curves that give it an S-shape, which makes it more shock-resistant. There are 33 vertebrae in all, of which there are three types (cervical, thoracic, and lumbar) in the spine, each type being of a different shape. Both the wedge-shaped sacrum and the tail-like coccyx at the base of the spine consist of fused vertebrae. Each vertebra is separated by disks of cartilage that cushion them from the stresses exerted by jumping, twisting, or weight-bearing.

CROSS SECTION OF SPINAL COLUMN

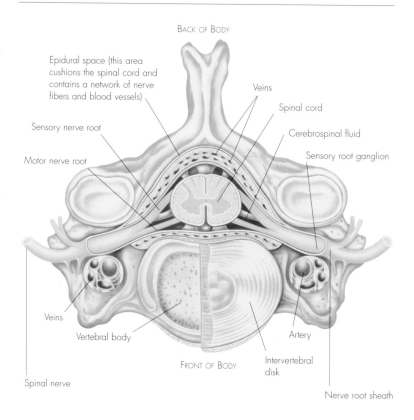

BACK OF BODY

Epidural space (this area cushions the spinal cord and contains a network of nerve fibers and blood vessels)

Veins

Spinal cord

Cerebrospinal fluid

Sensory nerve root

Sensory root ganglion

Motor nerve root

Veins

Vertebral body

Artery

FRONT OF BODY

Intervertebral disk

Spinal nerve

Nerve root sheath

A typical neck vertebra, seen from above. Note particularly the spinal cord and the spinal nerve roots.

Beneath the lumbar region there is the triangular sacrum, made up of five fused vertebrae and forming the back of the pelvis. The *coccyx*, a vestigial tail, is attached to the bottom of the *sacrum* and made up of four small vertebrae fused together. The sacroiliac joints (between the sacrum and the iliac bones in the pelvis) are critical to spinal function, transferring the movement and energy of the legs to the rest of the body.

The spine is not straight. It has several gentle curves, giving it an "S" shape. The cervical region is concave backwards; the thoracic region is convex backward;

and the lumbar region is again concave backward. This sinuous arrangement serves, among other things, to increase the shock-absorbing qualities of the spine.

Although no two vertebra are exactly alike, nearly all have the same general design. Each has a vertebral body, which is a more or less cylindrical mass of bone. Attached to the vertebral body at the back there is an arch of bone called the neural arch, which houses the spinal cord and other structures. Taken together the neural arches form the spinal canal, which houses the spinal cord. A vertebral spine projects backward from each neural arch; in a fairly slim person these spines can easily be felt through the skin in the thoracic region. Other pieces of bone project sideways from the neural arch; these are the transverse processes, to which muscles are attached. More pieces of bone, the articular processes, project upward and downward from each neural arch and interlock with the vertebrae immediately above and below, forming the facet joints. This arrangement contributes to the stability of the spine. However, a certain amount of bending and twisting movement is permitted; the range of movement is greatest in the neck and smallest in the lumbar region.

The vertebrae These are made of a special type of bone which has a hard outer covering while the interior is filled with a network of bone like a sponge. Bone of this kind contains red marrow, which makes the red cells of the blood and some of the white cells. Like other bones the vertebrae are covered with a special membrane called periosteum, which helps to nourish the bone and plays a part in repair after an injury such as a fracture.

The spinal joints

It is important to understand how the vertebrae are joined together because this has a bearing on back pain. There are two kinds of joints in the spine. The interlocking articular processes, which interlock above and below, between each vertebra, have synovial (facet) joints. These are similar to the joints found in many other parts of the body, such as the knee, and consist of surfaces covered with cartilage and surrounded by a special lubricating membrane (synovial membrane). Loss of or damage to this membrane can lead to various kinds of arthritis, which can affect the spine in the same way that they affect other joints.

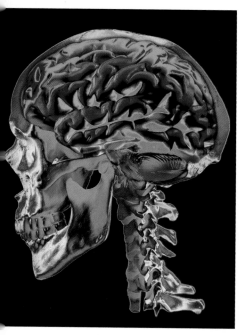

A side view of the skull and neck vertebrae. The neck vertebrae and muscles have to support the weight of the skull; the brain alone weighs just under 3 lb (1.4 kg).

The intervertebral disks The second kind of joint is found only in the spine. Each vertebral body is linked to the vertebrae above and below by a disk. This consists of a ring of tough fibrous tissue (the *annulus*) surrounding a jellylike core called the *nucleus pulposus*, which acts as a shock absorber. If a load is placed on the spine, when we are carrying a weight for example, the ring of fibrous tissue bulges a little, allowing the vertebrae to come a little closer to one another. This arrangement also allows the spine to bend in different directions and cushions the impact when we walk, run, and jump. There are considerable compressive forces on the intervertebral disks, and consequently we are a little taller in the morning than the evening, while astronauts, who are not subject to gravity, have been found to be as much as 4 in (100 mm) taller on their return to earth.

The notorious "slipped disk" is really due to the *nucleus pulposus* leaking out of the fibrous ring to compress neighboring structures such as nerves. Pain can also result from the release of irritating chemicals from the disk, even without a bulge. As we age, or if there is an injury, the *annulus* first develops a radial tear. The nucleus slides through the tear and causes a bulge in the *annulus*, which can cause pressure on either the posterior longitudinal ligament or the *dura mater* (see p. 21), either of which can cause significant back pain. If the bulge moves sideways, the portion of the *dura mater* that coats the nerve root becomes irritated, causing leg pain; there is neither weakness nor numbness at this point because the nerve itself is intact. If the annular bulge grows larger, or if the *annulus* ruptures and the *nucleus* escapes, the further increase in pressure that it then poses on the nerve root leads to loss of nerve function, which does cause leg weakness, numbness, or loss of reflex.

The disks have only a limited blood supply so healing after injury, if it occurs at all, is slow. Like other tissues, however, the disks do need oxygen, and for this they rely on diffusion (controlled leakage, in effect) of oxygen-rich fluid from the adjacent bones. The natural movement of the spine tends to increase diffusion, so mobility helps to keep the spine healthy – one reason why exercise is good for the back.

The skull

This is balanced on top of the spine, to which it is attached by two special vertebrae, the atlas and the axis. The atlas is the uppermost of these, and is named after the legendary giant in Greek mythology who carried the world on his shoulders. It is an approximately circular vertebra that lacks a true body; it has upward-facing facet joints that allow the head to make nodding movements. The axis is immediately

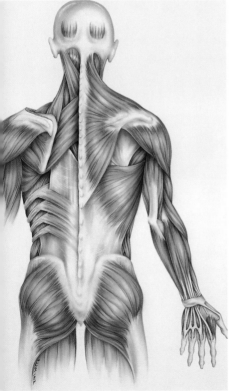

below the atlas and provides rotation (needed for turning movements).

The considerable weight of the skull is kept in place by a special peg of bone, a part of the axis, called the odontoid process. If the odontoid process is broken, as can happen in a severe whiplash injury or a fall, the atlas may slip and break the upper part of the spinal cord, causing immediate death. Because it is heavy, the skull exerts a lot of leverage on the neck vertebrae and this is one reason why pain may arise in this region.

The main muscles of the back are arranged in several layers. The most powerful muscles in the body are those that run along the spine, maintaining posture and providing strength. The upper back muscles that are attached to the scapula (shoulder blade) help stabilize the shoulder, the body's most mobile joint.

Ligaments and muscles

As well as the bones and joints, the spine has many ligaments holding it together. These are tough cords or sheets that bind the bones together, allowing a variable amount of movement between them. The ligaments in the lower back and pelvis are particularly strong. Although the ligaments are important, the stability of the spine also depends to a large extent on the numerous muscles that surround it; some of these are extremely strong, particularly those that begin at the pelvis and run up the spine to various levels. These muscles, together with their covering of connective tissue, are very important for keeping the spine in good condition.

But it is not only the muscles of the back that are important in this respect; so, too, are the abdominal muscles. These are involved in bending movements of the trunk, and they also increase the pressure inside the abdomen. This helps to prevent injury to the spine when lifting heavy weights; it is for this reason that weight lifters wear a belt. People with weak abdominal muscles or "potbellies" are at increased risk of disk injury. One pair of big muscles, the *psoas* muscles, are placed inside the abdominal cavity on its back wall and so cannot be seen or felt. They are attached to the upper part of the thighbone and so they act on the hip joint.

Like other muscles, the spinal muscles have a property called tone. This means that even when they are not contracting actively they are not completely relaxed but are always under slight tension. The amount of tone is set by nerve cells in the spinal cord and there is a feedback loop involving special sense organs in the muscles and tendons that constantly monitor the tone. Our ability to stand upright depends on the tone of the spinal and leg muscles. The spinal muscles hold the vertebral column up like the guy ropes on a tent. They keep us balanced, with the actual weight being supported mainly by the bones and ligaments. When we are standing, and even while walking, much of the sensation of fatigue arises from the ligaments rather than from the muscles. The muscles sometimes go into spasm, for example, to protect an injured vertebra; the spasm is caused by an increase in tone.

The spinal cord and nerves

A very important function of the spine is to protect the spinal cord, which is a projection downward from the brain and, like the brain, it contains numerous nerve pathways and nerve cells (neurons). At present, damage to the spinal cord, like

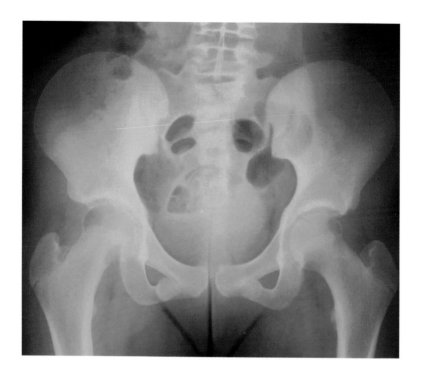

The pelvis is formed by the sacrum in the center and the two hipbones, and gives a strong structural foundation for the upper body.

damage to the brain, cannot be repaired, although recent experimental work suggests that this may become possible in the future. The spinal cord reaches as low as the upper border of the first lumbar vertebra in adults. Below this level the spinal canal houses a bundle of nerve roots called the *cauda equina* (horse's tail).

The spinal cord and brain have three layers of coverings. The innermost layer, the *pia mater*, is fine and delicate. Next comes the *arachnoid mater*, which is also quite delicate; the name means that it is like a spider's web. The third and outermost layer, the *dura mater*, is a tough sheath that protects the other layers and the underlying nerve tissue. They continue down the nerve roots as they leave the spinal cord.

The spinal nerves The way in which the spinal nerves emerge from the spinal cord is important. There are 31 pairs of spinal nerves, arranged in rows all the way down the cord; each nerve emerges from the spine through the gap between two adjacent vertebrae; this is called the intervertebral foramen. If for any reason the gap becomes smaller, perhaps because of arthritis or collapse of an intervertebral disk, the nerve may be squeezed and this can cause weakness, pain, or changes in sensation.

Each nerve is formed by the union of two nerve roots. The front (ventral) root is motor, supplying muscles; the rear (dorsal) root is sensory, carrying touch, heat and cold, pain, and so forth. The two roots unite to make a mixed nerve, motor and sensory. In some places several pairs of nerve roots unite to form a single large nerve; this is the case for the sciatic nerve, for example. The general arrangement of the spinal nerves is described as segmental; it is possible to relate particular areas of skin and particular muscles to the various spinal segments and this is useful in locating the level at which problems occur in the spine. For example, weakness and wasting of the small muscles in the hand indicate damage at the level of the upper thoracic or lower cervical regions, while pain in the big toe due to nerve compression must be coming from the lower lumbar or upper sacral nerve roots.

The autonomic nervous system

In addition to the motor and sensory nerves there is another type of nerves called the autonomic nervous system. This controls activities such as heart rate, glandular activity, intestinal movements, contraction and dilatation of the pupil; that is, activities that are not under voluntary control. It is customary to divide the autonomic nervous system into sympathetic and parasympathetic portions. The sympathetic part is mainly responsible for responses to emergencies. When we are threatened by danger we respond by preparing either to fight or to run away, and so we speed up our heart rate, increase the blood supply to our muscles, and so on. The parasympathetic part, in contrast, maintains those automatic functions such as digestion and relaxation that we rely on in the course of our ordinary activities. However, the distinction between these two kinds of function is not absolute and there is overlapping.

The pelvis

This is a bowl-shaped structure made up of the two hipbones and the *sacrum*. The sacroiliac joints, between the *sacrum* and the two pelvic bones, connect the legs to the spine. Unlike most, these joints move only very slightly. When we take a step, each joint acts by alternately transmitting force during weight bearing then, like a clutch, releasing it to allow the nonweight-bearing leg to swing forward.

At the same time, the attached ligaments – the largest and strongest in the body – store energy, which is released as each leg swings forward, and the spine itself twists, also storing energy. The sacroiliac joints are very rough and easily displaced, and if they become "stuck" in even a slightly abnormal position this whole process is disrupted, causing pain, stiffness, and reduced movement.

The joints between the *sacrum* and the two pelvic bones are unusual in that they allow only a small amount of movement. The legs are attached to the pelvis via the strong hip joints. The arms, in contrast, are not attached directly to the spine but are linked to it by muscles and, indirectly, by the clavicle (or collarbone) at the front of the neck. This means that the lower part of the spine is much more rigid than the upper part, which is an adaptation to our upright walking posture and the use of our hands for manipulating things.

Blood vessels

It is necessary for all these structures to be supplied with blood, and the back, therefore, contains many arteries and veins. Some of the structures do not have a rich blood supply, however, and healing, therefore, takes a long time if they are damaged; this applies to the ligaments and the intervertebral disks, for example. On the other hand, the vertebral bodies have a rich blood supply. Bone is of course a living tissue and this means that its shape can change, even in adults, in response to pressure. If a bone is subjected to stress it tends to become stronger; conversely, if it is not stressed at all, for example in patients confined to bed for long periods, it loses calcium and becomes weaker.

Individual variations

Everybody is unique and this applies to our anatomy, too. There may be individual variations in structure, some with important effects. Some people, for instance, have an extra rib in the neck (cervical rib), which may press on nerves or vessels; others have an extra lumbar vertebra, or vertebrae may be abnormally formed giving rise to symptoms. These anatomic anomalies are much more common in the lumbar spine than in the cervical spine. The tightness or laxity of people's ligaments can vary too.

symptoms
and their
causes

Accurately diagnosing diseases and conditions arising in or affecting the back can be complex. The symptoms that are produced are vital clues in determining, and therefore treating, the underlying cause. This section describes the different types of pain and other symptoms that people with back problems experience, and looks at the common, and some of the rarer, diseases and conditions that cause them.

Pain

Types of pain Many different kinds of symptoms can arise in the back but the most common is pain. In general terms there are three types of pain that can be felt anywhere in the body; all of these types of pain may occur in the back.

1 Pain with a specific identifiable cause: pain of this kind can arise either from the bones, muscles, joints , and connective tissue (burns, fractures, sprains), or from the internal organs (appendicitis, menstrual pain, etc.).

2 Pain due to nerve damage: this type of pain may be caused by nerve root compression or viruses; sometimes the cause is unknown. Pain of this kind is often

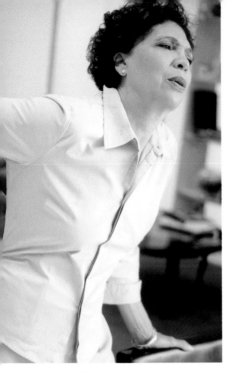

A sudden attack of back pain can strike anyone at any time.

called neuralgia. Examples are postherpetic neuralgia and trigeminal neuralgia. This kind of pain is often very severe and difficult to treat. Pain may also be caused by nerve injury or scarring as a result of surgery, and by reflex sympathetic dystrophy (RSD), which is also known as complex regional pain syndrome (CRPS), which causes sympathetic nerve pain and can result from many types of even minor injury; this pain is often severe and difficult to treat.

3 Chronic pain syndrome: some patients complain of widespread pain for no obvious reason; they "hurt all over." This is probably the most challenging kind of pain that practitioners have to deal with.

It is not always appreciated that we can to some extent separate the perception of pain from its emotional accompaniment. Thus, for a given level of pain one person may feel very distressed, while another remains stoic and "grins and bears it." This may be perceived as a "merely psychological" difference but in fact, these two pain components are processed by different mechanisms in the brain. One of the modern approaches to the management of pain consists of showing patients that it is possible to not be dominated by their pain.

Referred pain It is important to understand that the location of pain is not necessarily a guide to where the underlying problem is. In the case of pain arising from a motion segment (p. 27), for example, it is quite common for pain to be felt at some distance from the site of trouble. Many kinds of spinal disease do this, and the converse is also possible. That is, pain felt in the back may be coming from disease in another organ. This is known as referred pain. This is discussed in more detail on pp. 46–47.

Acute versus chronic pain Colloquially, people sometimes use these terms to refer to the severity of pain but, in fact, they refer to its duration. Acute pain means pain that comes on fairly suddenly, usually lasts for a definite, limited length of time, and then gets better. Chronic pain is pain that goes on for a long time with little tendency to get better, though its intensity may fluctuate. There is no fixed length of time that a pain must last before it is considered chronic, but as a rough guide one could say that pain lasting for more than three months has entered the chronic phase.

Many specialists think that chronic pain is a different disorder from the outset and is not simply acute back pain that failed to get better. It is true, however, that some patients will have recurrent back pain at intervals following an initial attack, though it is difficult to predict at the outset how likely this is to happen in any individual case. It is therefore sensible for anyone who has recovered from a first attack to follow the guidelines in the chapter on preventing back pain.

Subacute pain This term is sometimes used to refer to pain that is intermediate in duration between acute and chronic. In the case of the back, however, it is more appropriate to speak of "recurrent" pain, meaning pain that returns at intervals of months or years, although between attacks the patient is well.

Mechanical and nonmechanical pain

Another way of classifying back pain is by its causation. Here the broad categories are pain due to mechanical causes and pain due to systemic (widespread, affecting a number of body systems) disease . By mechanical pain we mean pain that is due to an identifiable cause such as a disk prolapse or a strained ligament. Nonmechanical pain is due to systemic disease such as rheumatoid arthritis or ankylosing spondylitis.

The distinction between these two categories is important because the treatment implications are different for the two types of pain. Mechanical back pain often responds to physical treatment such as manipulation, but this could be ineffective or even dangerous in pain due to a systemic disease. An important aim of diagnosis is therefore to exclude systemic disease even if identification of the exact nature of mechanical pain is not always possible.

Some causes of mechanical pain are fairly easy to diagnose because they show up on X-ray, a CT, or MRI scan (p. 51), or an injection of local anesthetic into tissue from which the pain is suspected to arise may confirm, or rule out, a diagnosis. However, this is not always the case. It has been known since the 1930s that many different tissues in the back can give rise to very similar types of back pain. For example, injecting an irritant-strength salt solution (hypertonic saline) into the back muscles and ligaments can cause radiation of pain and other sensations to the leg that is quite similar to sciatica (discussed in detail on pp. 36–37).

It is therefore not always possible to say with confidence exactly why a patient is suffering back pain. Such pain is sometimes ascribed to strained ligaments, trapped nerves, or minor displacements of joints (subluxation), but often these explanations, though plausible, lack direct proof.

Symptoms of mechanical back disorders

These can take many forms, not all of which are painful. Pain may be felt in the back itself or may radiate to the head, face, or limbs. The pain is often accompanied by joint stiffness, which is generally worse in the morning or after rest and improves with movement. Many patients also find that changes in the weather affect the severity and type of their symptoms.

The character of pain relates to its origin Many of the effects of these symptoms are difficult to explain in detail, but one way of classifying them is in relation to the structures from which they seem to originate. We can distinguish three main forms of pain (It is of course possible for a patient to have more than one of these types of pain):

1 Pain from a motion segment A "motion segment" consists of a pair of adjacent vertebrae and the joints between them, together with the muscles and ligaments in that region. This type of pain has a deep, dull, aching character and it may radiate to other areas in ways that are difficult to explain anatomically. For example, pain from the neck region may radiate to the top of the head or the eye; pain from the thoracic region may radiate to the front of the body; pain in the lumbar region may radiate to the lower abdomen, the buttock, or the foot. Clearly, radiation of this kind can make it difficult to diagnose the problem, especially if, as sometimes happens, there is no pain in the back itself.

2 Superficial pain Sometimes pain is felt in quite a localized area, for example over a particular spinous process. This type of pain affects skin and superficial muscles and ligaments. How it arises is not always clear but at times it seems to relate to the patient's posture. Bone pain is often localized and may result from direct trauma or ligament strain that, again, may be linked to posture.

3 Nerve compression pain This happens when a nerve root is compressed, for example as it emerges between two vertebrae. The pain is sharp in character and may feel like an electric shock (hitting one's "funny bone" produces a pain of this kind). Skin sensation may be impaired in the area supplied by the affected nerve and there may be weakness of muscles. Reflexes, such as the knee jerk, may be lost.

Other symptoms As well as pain, patients may complain of pallor or flushing, hearing disturbance and tinnitus, alterations of sensations in the face or scalp, and a feeling of a lump in the throat. There can be nausea and occasionally actual vomiting, difficulty in swallowing, feelings of pressure behind the eyes, and feelings of chest constriction. The alterations in sensations include "crawling" feelings in the scalp, heat, cold, and heaviness. These symptoms may be alarming and indeed it is possible that they might on occasion arise from serious diseases needing investigation and treatment, so it is important to mention them to the doctor. However, in many cases they are part of the back-pain picture, especially if the neck is involved. They are produced by changes in the functioning of the autonomic nervous system, which controls things like blood flow in the skin, swallowing, and the little muscle fibers that make one's hair "stand on end."

Spondylosis

Patients are often told that their back pain is due to "arthritis," which has the unfortunate implication that it is going to get progressively worse as time goes by. This is misleading in two ways: first, it is not necessarily true that symptoms will become worse as time goes by (they may even improve), and second, "arthritis" is only part of the story. There are several types of arthritis, the two common ones being rheumatoid arthritis and osteoarthritis.

Rheumatoid arthritis is a widespread disease affecting many joints throughout the body and tending to produce generalized symptoms such as anemia and weight loss. It often begins in the hands but later other joints may be affected, including the facet joints of the spine. The cause is unknown, but it belongs to the category of autoimmune diseases, in which the immune system of the body reacts against its own tissues. It can generally be diagnosed by blood tests. Although the spine may be affected, the disease is usually more evident in the limbs, and especially in the hands.

Osteoarthritis (also known as osteoarthrosis) affects particular joints, such as the knees, the hips, or the fingers (typically in women after menopause). In the spine it produces swelling and deformity of the small facet joints between the vertebrae.

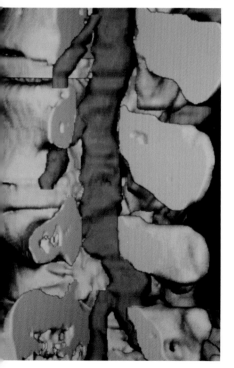

Although osteoarthritis is often ascribed to age and trauma, its cause is not clearly understood. It takes various forms, which may really be different diseases. One kind affects large joints such as the hip or knee, while another affects the small joints of the fingers, especially in women. In the back it affects the facet joints – the small synovial joints between the vertebrae. In osteoarthritis the articular cartilage (the "bearing surfaces" of the joints) becomes worn away until eventually there is

Here an intervertebral disk (in yellow, toward the bottom of the picture) has bulged out and is pressing on the spinal cord, which may give rise to symptoms of pain and weakness.

none left and the adjacent bone surfaces come into contact and rub against each other. This leads to pain, swelling, and loss of movement; eventually the joint may be almost totally destroyed.

In relation to back pain, osteoarthritis is only one part of the picture, which is why many doctors prefer to speak of "spondylosis." This includes osteoarthritis but covers other changes that also occur and that may be more important, such as the loss of disk space that tends to happen with age and that tends to place excessive loads on the facet joints, which can lead to osteoarthritis. We then have a chicken-and-egg situation in which it is difficult to say which is cause and which is effect.

Not all the changes of spondylosis are caused by osteoarthritis; some are due, for example, to degeneration of the disks. Osteoarthritis affects only synovial joints such as the facet joints, but there are other components of the spinal joints, such as the disks and ligaments as well as the bones, all of which are capable of causing pain. In this connection one tends to think of prolapsed disks (to be discussed shortly), but other disk abnormalities can occur as well. For example, disk material may escape upward or downward into the body of a vertebra, causing pain, or there may be loss of disk material with age, resulting in the vertebrae coming closer together and perhaps pressing on nerve roots. As a result of this loss of disk space there may be secondary degeneration in the facet joints of the spine. Patients need to understand that in this case disk surgery is unlikely to help their pain because it is really arising from the facet joints.

"Spondylosis," then, is a term that covers all the changes in the spine that occur with age and is therefore wider in scope than "osteoarthritis." While many doctors do use these terms separately, as described above, some use them interchangeably, which may cause confusion for the patient.

These changes with age are also sometimes referred to as "wear and tear," which is quite a good description. It is important to realize that spondylosis does not necessarily produce pain, and certainly there is no close connection between the severity of the changes as seen on X-ray and symptoms. You can have a lot of changes and little or no pain, or few changes and a lot of pain.

Spondylosis, or "wear and tear," is not a disease in itself. Changes in the structure and function of the spine are inevitable as we age, but the degree to which they give rise to symptoms is variable and unpredictable.

The rate at which spondylosis progresses is variable. Some people show changes sooner than others; indeed, they may occur even in the twenties, although symptoms generally appear a decade or two later. Partly this may be a question of heredity; osteoarthritis tends to run in families. But occupation also plays a part; hard labor causes osteoarthritic changes to appear in the spine and football players may have osteoarthritis of the knees, while gymnasts who enter competition too young may pay for it later in respect to their spines.

On X-ray, some people have evidence of osteophytes, which are outgrowths of bony tissue at the margins of the vertebral bodies. Although they look dramatic they do not cause pain unless they happen to compress a nerve root. In fact, by limiting spinal movement they may actually be protective to the spine.

Neck (cervical region) problems

The neck is one of the regions of the spine that commonly gives rise to pain, probably because of its mobility and the fact that the head exerts a lot of leverage in the neck structures. To get an idea of the amount of work the neck muscles have to do, take an 8 lb (4 kg) weight in your hand to represent your head and, with your elbow resting on a table, hold the weight vertically. Now try moving it around by bending your wrist, and you will get an idea of the strain on the muscles and joints in your neck. It is hardly surprising that this can cause problems from time to time.

Acute torticollis (wryneck) This affects mostly young people, especially teenagers. Typically the patient wakes up to find that his or her neck is painful and cannot be turned to one side. This disorder gets better by itself, with or without treatment, and usually in a few days, although it may take as long as 10 days. The cause is unknown, although one suggestion is that a nerve becomes pinched between two vertebrae while the patient is asleep. No specific treatment is needed apart from simple analgesics such as aspirin or acetaminophen if the pain is severe. It is possible that the duration of pain may be shortened by physical treatments such as acupuncture or manipulation but this has not been conclusively demonstrated in clinical trials.

Cervical spondylosis Wear and tear changes occur in the neck in practically everyone as they get older. They take the form of loss of intervertebral disk substance and degenerative changes in the facet joints. This form of neck pain thus mainly affects the middle-aged and elderly. As well as neck pain, there may be referred pain radiating down the arms or up into the head; there may be sensory changes, such as numbness or tingling, in the hands. Muscles in the hand may become weak if there is pressure on the nerves supplying them and, in severe cases, pressure on the spinal cord in the neck can cause symptoms including leg weakness and bladder problems.

Some elderly patients experience dizziness when they turn their head. There are many possible causes of such dizziness or vertigo, as it is termed, so it is important to get a diagnosis. One of the causes seems to be disease of the facet joints in the neck. We normally maintain our balance by a constant readjustment of muscle tone, and the complex computing system responsible for this relies on information about our position coming from a number of sources, including our eyes, the balance organs in our inner ears, and the special sense organs in our muscles and joints that tell us the positions of our limbs even when we are not looking at them. The facet joints in the neck are part of this system. They supply information about the position of the neck relative to the trunk, and this is important for the maintenance of balance. When these joints are distorted by osteoarthritis they may send abnormal messages that confuse the brain and interfere with its balance mechanism, so causing vertigo.

Neck pain due to spondylosis can take many forms. It may be present in the morning when the patient wakes up or it may come on later in the day in the course of activities such as driving or working at a desk. Typically the pain begins as a vague ache that becomes progressively worse as the day wears on. Later the pain spreads to other areas in the head, shoulder, or arm. Usually it is one-sided although sometimes both sides are affected. Pain of this kind is not always constant and unremitting; it often improves or even disappears after a few weeks or months although, unfortunately, it usually returns later.

Osteoporosis Many older people, women especially, suffer from osteoporosis. Loss of calcium from the bones makes them weak and the vertebrae may collapse, with a consequent increase in spinal curvature. In the neck this produces the so-called "dowager's hump," which is a bulge at the base of the neck. See p. 39 for more information on osteoporosis.

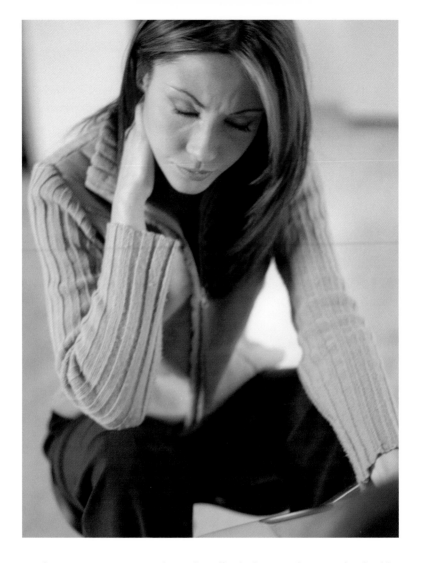

Neck tension causes pain in the neck itself, which can radiate into the shoulders or up into the head. It commonly affects young to middle-aged women.

Arthritis Any form of arthritis may affect the neck. Most often this is osteoarthritis, though in some cases it is rheumatoid arthritis (this is described in more detail in relation to spondylosis pp. 28–30).

Whiplash injury As road traffic increases, whiplash injuries have become increasingly common. It usually happens when a vehicle is hit from behind. The sudden shock moves the occupant's body forward but the head tends to stay still, so that the neck is violently flexed backward. There is then a reflex contraction of the neck's flexor muscles that coincides with the recoil of the neck into flexion, and it is during this phase that much of the damage is done. Seat belts do not help to prevent this kind of injury but properly adjusted headrests do. If the headrest is set too low, however, it may actually make matters worse, by forming a pivot round which the neck is bent. Whiplash injury can also occur in side impacts and in other kinds of accidents, such as diving.

In the immediate aftermath of a whiplash injury various symptoms may occur. The most common are neck pain and headache, but there may also be neck stiffness, shoulder pain, pain or numbness in the arms, pain in the face or throat, a feeling of numbness in the face, pain in the ears or eyes, problems with hearing or vision, a need to keep clearing the throat compulsively, vertigo, fatigue and depression, irritability, and sleep disturbance.

It is difficult to say what causes these symptoms. Some doctors have suspected that they are psychological or even in some cases are an attempt to get a good compensation settlement; however, symptoms often persist even after the claim has been settled and, indeed, may continue for months or years.

Immediately after a whiplash injury the patient must be assessed by a doctor to make sure that there is no dangerous instability of the spine caused by a fracture; in such cases urgent surgery may be required. First-aid workers take care not to move patients after an accident to prevent possible dislocation.

A great many treatments have been used in less severe cases, including use of an immobilizing collar, local heat and ice treatment, ultrasound, traction, massage, active and passive mobilization, pulsed electromagnetic therapy, and other multi-disciplinary methods. The fact that so many treatments have been tried makes it clear that there is no single answer to the problem but, the evidence suggests that patients should avoid using a soft collar and should remain active and try to return to their usual activities, if possible. Unfortunately, some people go on to suffer from chronic neck pain and this can be difficult to treat; manipulation or acupuncture help in some cases.

Some therapists use a device called a Photonic Stimulator to treat soft tissue damage including whiplash injury. This is a new device that has been approved for medical use by the FDA. It resembles a laser in producing a single wavelength of light (900 nm) but differs from a laser in that the light is not focused into a small beam.

Neck tension Probably the most common cause of neck pain is tension. The patient, who is often a woman in middle age or younger, experiences aching in the neck, usually more on one side. The pain may radiate to the shoulder, though seldom as far down as the hand, and there is no weakness or damage to the hand muscles. It may also radiate into the head, especially at the back, and patients may describe this as a headache. In some people the front of the head is affected, with pain in the forehead and eyes; this sometimes leads to a mistaken diagnosis of chronic sinusitis. Neck movements are usually limited and there is frequently tenderness of the neck and shoulder muscles, which feel more tense than usual.

The cause of this kind of pain is difficult to establish. Often, though not always, patients recognize that there is a definite connection between their symptoms and their psychological state, which is frequently one of mild depression or anxiety. However, treatment with psychotherapy or antidepressants does not usually help much. Physical treatments such as manipulation or acupuncture may be more successful although they seldom provide a permanent cure. An interesting finding is that massage, acupuncture, or manipulation can sometimes trigger an emotional reaction, in which the patient may laugh or cry for quite a long time without knowing why; it is as if their emotions had somehow become locked into their physical state and were then released by the treatment.

Postural neck pain As in other regions of the spine, pain can arise as a result of poor posture. Common causes here include constantly keeping the head thrust forward — in front of a computer terminal, for example — and clamping the phone between shoulder and neck. (See "Preventing Back Pain" p. 69.)

Chest (thoracic region) problems

On the whole this region is probably less commonly a site of pain than either the neck or the lumbar region, but pain may nevertheless occur here. One likely cause is postural. The patient is often a middle-aged woman who complains of constant aching across the shoulders and in the upper back; arm movements are restricted so that lifting objects off a shelf or hanging up clothes are difficult. These patients have a considerable degree of fixity in the upper part of the thoracic spine, the shoulders are rounded, and the upper part of the spine and the ribs move hardly at all. Physiotherapy to increase the range of movement may be helpful for such patients.

Pain originating in the thoracic spine may be referred to other areas, notably the front of the chest where it may be confused with heart pain (angina). Pain referred from the lower part of the thoracic spine can refer pain to the abdomen, where it may suggest disease of internal organs.

Disease of the thoracic vertebrae may occasionally cause pressure on the spinal cord — this is similar to pressure on the cord occurring in the neck and can give rise to weakness of the legs or bladder-emptying problems. Fortunately, however, this is rare. Urgent referral to a surgeon is needed in such cases.

Lower-back (lumbar region) problems

This is probably the region of the spine where pain most often arises. Two terms are commonly used to describe this kind of pain: "lumbago" means an ache in the lower back; "sciatica" should strictly mean pain in the areas supplied by the sciatic nerve but is often used more loosely to mean any pain that radiates down the leg.

Sciatica Sciatica may begin relatively abruptly or gradually. One common way for it to start is after an unusual exertion, such as digging the garden for the first time after the winter or bending over to lift a car tire when repairing a flat. Sometimes the initial stress is quite minor, for example stepping off a curb. Immediately after the stress the patient feels some lumbar aching but this is usually mild. But within a day or two the pain becomes more severe and the back muscles go into spasm, so that the back is stiff and the patient is unable to bend forward. This is a protective spasm by the muscles to prevent movement and therefore limit further damage.

Shortly after this the pain shifts from the back to one or other buttock and begins to radiate down the leg; at this point the spasm in the back muscles often eases off. The leg may feel cold as well as painful and there may be other strange sensations such as pins and needles. There may be areas in the leg where sensation is lost and certain muscle groups may be weak. When your doctor tests your reflexes these may be weak or absent. This state lasts for several weeks and then recovery usually begins.

Other types of sciatic pain It is possible for pain down the leg to come from other structures in the lumbar region. One of these is the sacroiliac joint at the back of the pelvis. Exactly how this happens is uncertain, though one theory is that the joint becomes slightly out of place (subluxated), perhaps for postural reasons or after childbirth. Strain on the ligaments is another possible cause; manipulation or acupuncture may help with pain coming from this area. Yet another possible site of pain is the muscles in the buttock that act on the hip joint (as in the rare piriformis syndrome), which may have tender areas called trigger points (see p. 44) or, according to one theory, may entrap the sciatic nerve. In all these cases, however, muscle wasting and loss of sensation do not occur; this helps in making the diagnosis. It is important to distinguish these types of "sciatica" from those that are due to disk pressure on nerves, because if disk prolapse is present manipulation may make matters worse, while in other types it can help.

Lumbar disk prolapse ("slipped disk") Probably most people think at once of a "slipped disk" in relation to lumbago and sciatica, but this is by no means always the cause of pain of this kind. As explained in the Structure chapter (see p.18), disks cannot slip. What happens is that the soft material (nucleus pulposus) in the center of the disk leaks out (prolapses) into the spinal canal and presses on the adjacent nerve roots. The prolapse may occur centrally or to either side. The pressure on the nerve root leads to pain, often combined with weakness of the muscles supplied by that nerve and to areas of sensory loss. The distribution of these symptoms allows the doctor to localize the level of the trouble in the spine with reasonable accuracy. In most cases recovery occurs over a period of a few weeks. If the symptoms persist it may be necessary to consider some form of intervention such as surgery. Disk prolapse can occur at any level in the spine but is most common in the lumbar region.

Neurogenic claudication In contrast to sciatica, a different type of leg pain referred from the back is due to narrowing of the spinal canal in the lumbar region, for example by spondylosis. This is neurogenic claudication, meaning limping due to nerve damage. There may be uncomfortable sensations in the legs, which patients describe as numbness, coldness, burning, or cramp. What is distinctive about this disorder is that the symptoms come on when patients stand upright, especially when they walk, and disappear when they bend forward. Cycling may be comfortable although walking is painful. The disorder is rather similar to intermittent claudication, which is much more common and is due to narrowing of the leg arteries. One point of difference between the two is that patients with intermittent claudication prefer to walk downhill because it is less demanding, whereas patients with neurogenic claudication prefer to walk uphill because then they are leaning forward.

Chronic stress backache This type of backache affects men more than women, especially strongly built stocky men with a protuberant abdomen who are used to performing heavy work (the typical beer belly type). These patients complain of pain in the middle and lower back that radiates to the flanks, buttocks, and groin, but without sciatica. This kind of pain begins gradually and eventually becomes almost continuous. The cause of the pain is unclear but may be ligamentous strain.

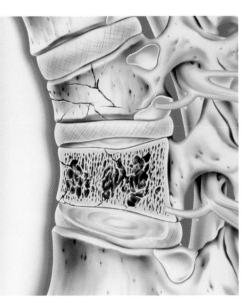

Spondylolisthesis This refers to slipping forward of a lumbar vertebra. The lumbar spine is normally curved forward (normal lordosis); the weight of the body tends to force the vertebrae forward but this is normally prevented by the ligaments of the spine and by the shape of the facet joints. However, weakness of a vertebra, which may be congenital or due to wear and tear, may

The middle vertebra in this illustration shows the spongy nature of the bone in this region. The uppermost vertebra, shown here with cracks on its surface, has collapsed due to osteoporosis.

allow the body of the vertebra to separate from the rest of the bone and slip forward. A single severe injury may have the same effect. There may be no symptoms at all and the condition may be found incidentally on an X-ray or CT scan; if symptoms do occur they may take the form of low back pain radiating into the legs together with tenderness of the affected vertebra. Research indicates that injury during adolescence is a common cause of spondylolisthesis, and treatment depends on the type of problem resulting from the slipped vertebra.

Osteoporosis

Osteoporosis affects everyone to some extent as they age but is particularly troublesome in postmenopausal women. It is due to progressive loss of calcium from the body. The result is that the bones become weaker and may eventually break even with quite minor injuries. The common sites for fractures are the hip and the vertebrae, which tend to collapse and become wedge-shaped. The affected vertebra may be painful and there may also be referred pain owing to pressure on nerve roots. As more vertebrae collapse the patient tends to lose height and may develop a "dowager's hump." There may be pain in the back even though no fracture has occurred.

For more information about preventing osteoporosis please refer to p. 73, and p. 108 for information about its treatment.

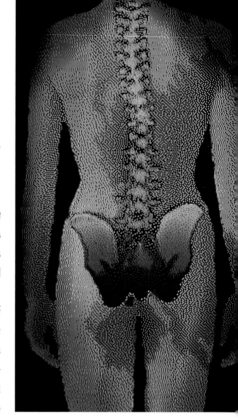

Scoliosis: the spine is bending sideways to the right in the the lower thoracic and upper lumbar regions. There is also an element of twisting.

Other diseases and conditions

Scoliosis This is a twisting of the spine. It may be secondary, caused by other diseases affecting muscles or nerves. Primary scoliosis occurs as a separate disease; there are several types, all of which affect the growing spine.

Idiopathic scoliosis, meaning scoliosis of unknown cause, occurs in children or adolescents. The best-known form affects mainly adolescent girls and is seen in the mid-thoracic spine, which is nearly always convex to the right. The deformity becomes more obvious if the child is asked to touch her toes. It does not clear up by itself and indeed it may become worse with time, so X-rays are taken every few months to monitor progress. Physiotherapy, perhaps with the addition of a brace, may prevent deterioration; sometimes a plaster cast or traction is required, and occasionally, surgery is needed.

Another type of scoliosis, more common in Europe than in America, affects boys more than girls and occurs before the age of three. It clears up by itself in over half the cases; if it does not, a corrective splint may be applied; rarely, surgery is performed when the child is about 10 years old.

A third type of scoliosis is described that affects children aged between four and nine years; it seems to be a mixture of the two preceding types.

Vertebral fracture Vertebrae may be fractured by trauma in the same way as other bones, even if there is no osteoporosis. A fall, especially on the buttocks, can cause a vertebral body to collapse, while other fractures affect the vertebral arch and separate the body from the arch. Occasionally a strong muscular contraction may break off a transverse process to which the muscle is attached. No treatment is generally given for such fractures apart from pain-relieving medication, and healing will usually occur naturally. The main exception to this is in the upper cervical region where instability of the vertebrae is potentially dangerous and surgery may be needed. Kyphoplasty is being used more often in the United States for treating vertebral fractures. Plastic is injected into the disk to maintain its height. Sometimes a balloon is inserted and then inflated. Injury to the *coccyx* may cause severe pain. Some people, usually women, suffer severe pain in the *coccyx* without any history of injury. The cause of this pain is obscure and it is often difficult to help, although some therapists find photonic stimulation to be beneficial.

Schuermann's disease (vertebral osteochondrosis) Like idiopathic scoliosis, this disorder usually occurs in youth and affects principally teenagers. It is thought to be due to the nuclear pulp within an intervertebral disk projecting into an adjacent vertebral body through a defect. It may cause little trouble, but sometimes it leads to severe disturbance of growth and causes kyphosis of the spine ("hunchback").

Arachnoiditis The arachnoid membrane is the middle of the three coverings of the brain and spinal cord. Arachnoiditis means an inflammation of the arachnoid membrane. It used to occur after an oil-based insoluble fluid was injected into the spinal canal to show it up in X-rays. Modern methods of imaging have rendered this unnecessary but arachnoiditis still occurs at times after operations on the spine, after infections, or for unknown reasons. It does not always cause symptoms but it can give rise to persistent pain that is difficult to treat. It may clear up without treatment.

Paget's disease of bone This is a disease of unknown cause, though it may be due to a virus. Areas of bone are destroyed and then repaired and the affected bone may become thicker as a result. It can affect any bones, including the vertebrae, but it is particularly common in the lumbar spine, skull, and pelvis. There may be no symptoms at all or it may cause persistent pain. There is no cure; pain-relieving drugs are used as necessary and acupuncture can help some patients.

Gout Many people think of gout as affecting only the big toe, but it can also involve other joints including those of the spine. It is due to high levels of uric acid in the blood and is not, contrary to popular belief, necessarily caused by an over-indulgent lifestyle. At the same time as pain in their toes or other joints, patients may experience severe backache to such a degree that it is almost impossible to move. Gouty patients seem particularly liable to suffer painful osteoarthritis of the spine. Effective drugs exist to lower the uric acid level in the blood and this prevents acute attacks and progressive deterioration of the joints and kidneys.

Polymyalgia rheumatica This is an important if not very common cause of back pain that affects mainly the hip and shoulder regions. It is important both because it is easily treated once diagnosed and also because it is associated with temporal arthritis, which can cause sudden blindness if untreated. Women are affected by polymyalgia rheumatica more than men and the disease usually occurs after the age of 60. It can come on very quickly and is characterized by severe muscle pain. Treatment is with corticosteroids (prednisolone), which keep the disease under control until it clears up spontaneously, which it generally does after some months or years.

Ankylosing spondylitis This is a type of arthritis that is more common in men than in women. There is a tendency for it to run in families because it is linked to a particular genetic trait. It causes stiffness of the spine as well as pain and in severe cases the spine may become completely rigid, though many patients have only mild symptoms. Anti-inflammatory drugs can help to control pain and patients are encouraged to remain as mobile as possible. Acupuncture affords pain relief for some patients though it does not alter the progression of the disease.

Reiter's disease This is an inflammation of the spine that may (rarely) follow an attack of urethritis. Other joints, such as the knees, are often involved, too. Treatment depends on the symptoms, and involves medication and perhaps acupuncture.

Shingles (*herpes zoster*) This is one form of what is called neuropathic pain, meaning pain due to nerve damage. It is due to reactivation of the chicken pox virus, left over from a chicken pox illness that probably occurred many years previously. The virus takes up residence in the nerve cells in the sensory roots of the spinal cord. Later, when immunity is reduced for some reason such as old age or being "run down," the virus may become active again, usually in just one nerve. It does not cause chicken pox this time but it does cause a rash on the skin over the area of the body supplied by the nerve root in question. There is usually a period of backache for about seven to ten days before the rash appears and the diagnosis can be difficult to make at this time. When the rash appears it takes the form of blisters that quickly burst to become small pustules, and the skin in the affected region is inflamed and very sensitive. After the pustules heal an area of scarring remains.

Shingles most frequently appears on the chest but it may also occur on a limb or on the face; if the eye is involved, expert treatment from an eye specialist is needed to prevent damage to sight. Very occasionally the rash does not appear at all and occasionally, it affects both sides of the body. There is no truth in the old superstition that it is fatal if the rash meets in the middle. Because shingles is a reactivation of the virus rather than a new infection, being near children with chicken pox does not put older people at risk of shingles.

The amount of pain and the severity of the rash are variable. The worst feature of shingles is that it may leave the patient suffering from a chronic pain syndrome, called postherpetic neuralgia. The risk of this happening is greater the older the patient. Early treatment may reduce the risk of this complication, so older sufferers should see their doctor as soon as possible. Fortunately, once someone has suffered one attack of shingles it is unlikely that they will experience another.

Cancer Although this is by no means a common cause of back pain the doctor always has to keep the possibility in mind when seeing a middle-aged or elderly patient in whom the symptoms persist. Tumors of various organs, such as the lung, thyroid, kidney, breast, and prostate are especially liable to cause secondary tumors in the spine, and other forms of cancer such as multiple myeloma may begin there.

Infections It is rare for infections to settle in the spine. Bacteria from a urinary tract infection or other source may cause an abscess in the spine, especially when resistance is reduced, perhaps by diabetes. At one time tuberculosis of the spine was quite common, especially in children. It has now become rare but the recent increase of tuberculosis means that we may begin to see more of it. Modern anti-tubercle drugs avoid the need for the prolonged periods in plaster cast splints that used to be required for healing.

Trigger point disorders

Trigger points are tender areas, mainly in muscles, from which pain and other sensations radiate to distant areas. Their existence is not recognized by everyone and doctors do not usually learn about them during their training; however, they seem to be quite a real phenomenon. Many practitioners now believe that they are a very important cause of pain and disability. Trigger point disorders are increasingly becoming familiar to physiotherapists, osteopaths, and chiropractors who work with problems of the muscles and joints.

Almost everyone has a few latent trigger points that do not cause any symptoms. They can become active in various ways. Common causes are injury, sudden strains, undue exertion, and emotion. Any unusual activity, such as lifting a heavy weight awkwardly or taking up a new sport too energetically, may set them off. Once activated they can persist for long periods, giving rise to pain and other effects such as weakness or circulation changes. Common sites for trigger points are the neck and shoulder muscles, where they can cause headaches and other kinds of head pain, and the low back and gluteal region, where they cause symptoms suggesting sciatica.

It is possible to inactivate trigger points in various ways, ranging from simple pressure with the fingers to acupuncture or injection of local anesthetic or corticosteroids into the trigger points. Once this has been achieved the trigger point itself may become inactive and the areas of pain that it was causing may disappear.

Two main types of trigger point disorder are recognized. One is fairly localized and is known as the myofascial pain syndrome. This kind may have a definite cause, such as a sudden strain, and often responds well to treatment. The other kind is more widespread and is known as fibromyalgia.

Fibromyalgia This is a disorder that mainly affects women. They complain of constant, often incapacitating, pain, mainly in the trunk (thoracic and lumbar regions) and also feel generally unwell. Blood tests show nothing amiss, which is one way of making the important distinction from polymyalgia rheumatica. On examination one finds a great many trigger points in their back muscles, far more than in a typical case of myofascial pain syndrome (pain affecting muscles and tissues, more localized than fibromyalgia). There is usually sleep disturbance and

---

Increased lordosis (hollow in the lumbar region) in pregnancy causes strain on the joints of the lower back, and may cause backache. Softening of the spinal ligaments is also a contributing factor.

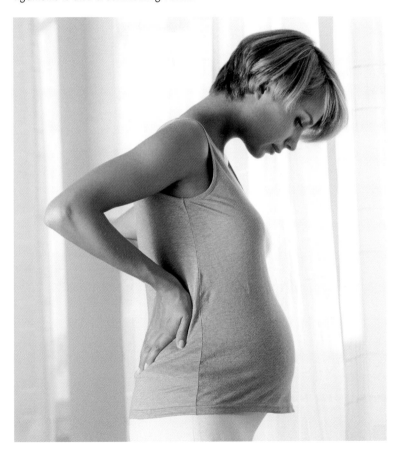

patients wake up feeling tired. Ordinary pain-relieving medicines such as aspirin, acetaminophen, and NSAIDs (nonsteroidal anti-inflammatory drugs) have little effect on the pain. Antidepressants are often used and sometimes seem to help; this is both because the patients are, in fact, often depressed, and also because the drugs have some pain-relieving properties in their own right. The cause of fibromyalgia is unknown. It seems to be part of a group of disorders that include chronic fatigue syndrome.

Backaches in pregnancy

It is common for pregnant women to get backaches and there is a tendency to dismiss it as unimportant or even "normal", but it is important for pregnant women to understand why it occurs and what they can do to reduce it.

There are several causes for backache in pregnancy. The weight of the uterus and its contents places extra strain on the back, forcing the woman to lean back. This increases the normal hollow in the lumbar region (lordosis). During pregnancy a hormone called relaxin is secreted that softens the ligaments of the pelvis, which makes the pelvic joints more liable to move, thus facilitating childbirth. Pain referred from the sacroiliac joints is felt typically in the buttocks and thighs.

Though these are ample causes for backaches, other factors may be involved. Joint laxity may cause vertebrae to slip forward (spondylolisthesis). Although pregnancy does not usually cause disk prolapse, it may make a preexisting prolapse worse, and there also seems to be an increased tendency for prolapse to occur after pregnancy.

Backaches usually improve after delivery, but not always, and sometimes they come on for the first time after delivery. Epidural anesthesia is often blamed for this, but research suggests that it is not responsible. Probably what happens is that, when questioned after some months or years, women forget that they had backaches during the pregnancy and think that it came on only after delivery, and therefore attribute it to the anesthetic.

Pain referred to the back

Not only may pain be referred from the back, but various organs may refer pain to the back. In other words, pain felt in the back may be coming from somewhere else.

There are certain danger signs in back pain that, if they are present, should prompt a visit to the doctor. Recent onset of back pain in someone over 50 or under 20 needs to be investigated. Pain that is much worse at night or when lying down is another danger sign. Attention is also needed if the pain is accompanied by constitutional symptoms such as weight loss, fever, or chills, or if the patient is at risk for a spinal infection because of a recent infection such as a boil or urinary tract infection, or suffers from diabetes. A history of intravenous drug abuse or of taking drugs that suppress the immune system is also important.

This is a result of the way the nerve supply to the organs is distributed from the spinal cord. Each organ is linked to a particular level or segment of the cord, and disease in that organ can cause pain to be felt in the back at the corresponding level. As a rule, the pain is also felt in the organ, but sometimes it is felt only in the back and diagnosis can then be difficult.

Causes of referred back pain Ulcers in the stomach or duodenum may refer pain to the back. The original site of trouble may be identified if the pain is worse after swallowing acidic foods such as fruit, and better when drinking milk or taking antacid medicine. Disease of the pancreas often causes back pain as can gall-bladder and colon disease.

Kidney disease frequently causes referred pain to the lower back as can prostate disease in men.

An important although fortunately rare type of back pain is caused by an abdominal aortic aneurysm. The aorta is the largest artery in the body and it runs down inside the abdomen, where it rests against the spine. In older people the aorta may become dilated; this is an aneurysm. If, as sometimes happens, pain is the only symptom, this may lead to delay in diagnosis. If an elderly patient who is taking anticoagulants (which slow blood clotting) – such as warfarin or aspirin – experiences a sudden onset of back pain, it may indicate that there has been bleeding into the back wall of the abdomen. The patient should be seen immediately by a doctor.

diagnosis

Diagnosis refers to the process of trying to find out what is causing a patient's symptoms. It can often be difficult to reach a firm conclusion about this because the back is such a complicated structure. However, there is also an important negative aspect to diagnosis, which consists in ruling out serious disease. The main question is whether the pain is "mechanical," in which case it may well cure itself, or is a manifestation of some possibly serious underlying disease

When to call your doctor

As a rule there is no need to see your doctor immediately if you are suffering acute back pain. The main exceptions to this advice are if there is any disturbance of bladder or bowel function, or if there is severe sciatica, especially with weakness of the leg. If the back pain is very severe and does not respond to bedrest or simple painkillers, that would also be a reason to call your doctor.

Medical examination If you do see your doctor, the main emphasis in the consultation will probably be on making sure that none of the "red flag" features, suggesting a systemic disease, are present. The doctor will take a history and probably carry out a physical examination, which will vary according to the circumstances. The doctor will check your range of movements and press on your spine to check for local tenderness. If you are a middle-aged or elderly man your prostate may be checked. Your leg strength and tendon reflexes will be tested. On the basis of all this the doctor will probably be able to make at least a provisional diagnosis and will provide treatment to control your pain, as well as advice about how much movement you should undertake and when you are likely to be able to resume your normal activities.

RED FLAG SYMPTOMS

- Possible fracture
- A recent severe fall or accident
- A recent minor accident in someone with a vulnerable spine, such as a patient with osteoporosis
- Constitutional symptoms (fever, chills, weight loss)
- Recent onset of pain in someone over 50 or under 20
- Possible infection or cancer
- Risk factors for spinal infection (recent infection, especially urinary infection; intravenous drug abuse; diabetes; drugs that suppress the immune system
- Pain that is much worse when the patient is lying down; severe nighttime pain
- Cauda equina syndrome (pressure on nerve roots in lower lumbar region):
- Recent onset of bladder problems
- Severe or progressive weakness of legs
- Loss of sensation in lower back or perineum

The value of X-rays? There is seldom any need to undertake any investigations at this stage unless there is reason to suspect some more serious underlying disease. Patients sometimes ask whether they should have an X-ray, but this is unlikely to be helpful in most cases. True, it may show "disk space narrowing," but by itself this does not mean much. It indicates that some disk material has escaped at some time but this may well be irrelevant to the present pain episode. It may show other features, such as osteoarthritic changes in the facet joints, but these again are not of much help in diagnosis.

Since it is generally desirable to reduce exposure to X-rays as much as possible they are not usually carried out in cases of acute back pain. The main exceptions are if a fracture, perhaps due to osteoporosis, or cancer are suspected. In other words, X-rays in back pain are done mainly to rule things out rather than to provide a definite diagnosis. When it is thought desirable to look for disk prolapse or "trapped nerves," more sophisticated methods, such as MRI or CT scans (see p. 51) are generally used today.

Chronic and recurrent back pain

Some people experience just one attack of acute back pain in their lives and never have another. At the other extreme some unfortunates are in more or less continuous pain (chronic), although its severity may vary. In between episodes some have recurring back pain at intervals while remaining more or less pain-free at other times.

Acute and chronic pain are different in many ways although there is a degree of overlap. Some of the investigations and treatments that are generally used for chronic (long-term) pain are sometimes also used in a first acute attack, particularly if it is severe.

The small number of people who do not recover quickly from acute back pain – perhaps after three months – may be referred to a specialist. Sometimes a specialist may be seen earlier during the acute phase, for example if the pain is very severe or if there is significant sciatica. (see pp. 36–37)

Many patients expend much time, effort, and money in an attempt to find a mechanical cause for chronic back pain such as a "slipped disk" (disk prolapse), a tear of an annular ligament, spondylolisthesis, or spinal canal narrowing, but this is a quest that can be taken too far. Often nothing abnormal is found after investigations, and even if it is, it may not be relevant to the patient's symptoms. MRI scans (see p. 51) may show reduced spinal movements, "wear and tear" changes in the spine, osteoarthritis of facet joints, or abnormalities of the disks and even disk protrusions, but these things seldom have any close relation to the symptoms the patients complain of.

Also, severe symptoms can occur without any abnormalities showing up in the investigations. What all this amounts to is that much skill and judgment are required to interpret the results of the sophisticated tests that are available today, and it has to be accepted that, even with the help of these tests, an identifiable "cause" that can be remedied will not always be found.

There have been many studies of back pain sufferers. These have shown little connection between back problems and people's height or weight. Spinal deformity, unless very severe, does not seem to be relevant, nor do differences in spinal movements or muscle strength. Disk degeneration shown on X-ray does not seem to be significant either.

Specialist diagnosis (CT and MRI scans)

The specialist, who may be either a neurosurgeon or an orthopedic surgeon, will take a history and carry out a physical examination in much the same way as your GP, though perhaps in more detail. Some blood tests will probably be ordered to rule out systemic disease. An X-ray will probably not be done because there is little connection between the amount of pain a patient feels and any changes that may appear on an X-ray. In any case, more sophisticated investigations are now available. There have been remarkable advances in "imaging" in recent years; that is, in the ability to see inside the living body and picture what is going wrong.

The two main techniques are CTs (computerized tomography) or MRIs (magnetic resonance imaging). These have largely replaced myelography, in which a fluid opaque to X-rays was injected into the spine to outline the spinal cord and nerve roots, and have also mostly replaced radiculography, which was the standard method until recently but is now carried out only if an MRI is not available.

CT scan An ordinary X-ray shows all the structures in one overlapping plane, so that they may be difficult to distinguish from one another. For this reason two films are usually taken, at right angles to each other. Another disadvantage with a plain X-ray is that it does not show up the soft tissues (muscles, nerves, disks, and so on) in any detail. Tomography was introduced to overcome these difficulties, by taking a number of films at slightly different angles and then combining the resultant images.

With the development of fast computers it has become possible to construct very detailed images that show the interior of the body in a three-dimensional representation. Although X-rays are used in this technique the dosage is fairly low. The CT is the best method of showing bone abnormalities and will also detect lesions of disks and other soft tissues.

MRI scan This is the best method of showing soft tissue lesions such as disk prolapse but is still not available everywhere. In an MRI, the patient is placed in a very strong magnetic field that cannot be felt. It causes the nuclei of the atoms in the body to line themselves up in a particular orientation; when the magnetic field is switched off they lose this orientation and the rate at which they do so is measured.

Different tissues lose orientation at different rates and this difference is measured to allow a picture of the internal structures to be constructed.

Like CTs, MRIs can produce very striking images of the interior of the body. This has made a dramatic difference in the diagnosis of back pain, but the very success of the technique has created its own issues of interpretation. Many people show some degree of abnormality on MRI scanning but this may not be causing any symptoms. Therefore, both MRI and CT scans need to be carefully interpreted, and only those findings that match up with the patient's clinical symptoms should be used to guide treatment.

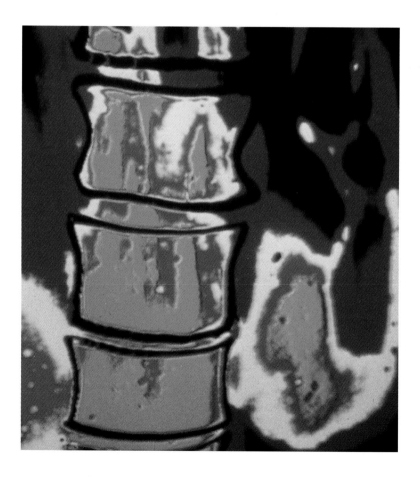

Other investigations

In addition to first-line methods of investigation (CT, MRI) others such as discography, bone scans, and electromyography may have an important role to play in getting to the root of some back problems.

Discography This is performed by injecting, under pressure, a liquid opaque to X-rays, directly into the intervertebral disks. This is done to determine whether or not the disks are the source of pain. When normal disks are injected there is no pain; when a diseased disk is injected the patient's pain is reproduced. This also isolates which disk is causing the problem and enables appropriate treatment to be planned.

Bone scans These are performed by injecting a radioisotope; this is done if bone disease, such as multiple myeloma, is suspected.

Electromyography (EMG) This s a painful procedure involving the insertion of fine needles into the muscles to record their electrical activity. It is used only to clarify a difficult diagnosis. EMG is used to show interruptions in nerve conduction, or an irritation; it can confirm nerve root involvement, and can detect peripheral nerve entrapment, such as carpal tunnel syndrome, causing numbness and/or pain in the limbs.

Risk factors for back pain

Perhaps surprisingly, the factors that do seem to be important are not directly related to the back. They include: disease of the heart and lungs, smoking, depression, poor work conditions,social class, lack of education, and poverty.

Smoking The connection with diseases of the heart and lungs and with smoking is relatively easy to explain. Smoking causes atherosclerosis (narrowing of the arteries). If the spinal arteries that supply blood to the disks are narrowed, the disks tend to degenerate. Smoking also reduces the amount of oxygen delivered by red

MRI scans can show the detailed structure of the spine in the living back.

blood cells to the disks and this, too, causes disk degeneration. The damaged disks may not press on nerve roots directly to produce the classic signs of sciatica, but they may cause problems in other ways. They may place strain on the facet joints or on ligaments (see Spondylosis, pp. 28–31) and this can cause pain. They can also compress the epidural veins. This leads to damage to the nerve roots and, by a cascading effect, to inflammation in the blood vessels in the spine and so to further damage. And the disks themselves can become painful and sensitive. One or several levels of the spine may be affected in this way, but the changes cannot easily be seen with existing methods of imaging such as MRIs or CTs.

Depression The connection with psychological disorders such as depression should not, of course, be taken to mean that chronic back pain is "all in the mind." Whatever their ultimate cause or causes, psychological disorders are themselves manifestations of alterations in brain function. And it is becoming increasingly understood that much, and perhaps all, chronic pain, is linked to changes in the way that the brain processes pain. For example, a particular part of the center of the brain called the anterior cingulate cortex (the site where physical and psychological influences interact) is abnormally active in patients suffering from a certain kind of pain in the face called atypical facial pain. Whether this is also true of chronic back pain is unknown but seems quite likely.

A holistic approach to diagnosis

All this means that, in trying to diagnose chronic back pain and how best to treat it, many factors have to be taken into account. Patients are sometimes puzzled, disappointed, and even resentful when they are told that the cause of their back pain may not be in the back itself and may be related to their circumstances or psychological state, but this is a necessary consequence of recognizing the complex interactions that exist between the muscles and joints on the one hand and the central nervous system (spinal cord and brain) on the other.

Ultimately, pain is produced within the brain and is a consequence of certain patterns or pathways becoming activated. This can happen as a result of changes in the muscles and joints but it can also happen in other ways, including changes that take place entirely within the brain itself. A good example of this is phantom

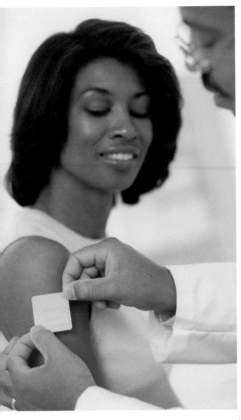

Nicotine patches are one of a range of aids now available to help people give up smoking, a risk factor for back pain.

limb pain. After a limb is amputated the patient may continue to feel severe pain in the missing limb. Clearly this has to be due to events within the brain. Something rather similar seems to underlie a good deal of chronic back pain. It is not useful to argue about whether such pain is "psychological" or "physical"; it is both.

The following analogy may also help. Suppose you are starting to print out something on your computer and the printer suddenly comes to a halt. In terms of the analogy this is equivalent to an episode of back pain. There are various possible causes. Some are within the printer itself; you may have a paper jam, for example. This would correspond to a mechanical back problem such as a strained ligament or a vertebral fracture. The lead connecting your computer to your printer might have come loose; this corresponds to pressure on a nerve root leading to weakness of muscles and loss of sensation. You could have acquired a computer virus; this corresponds to a biological virus such as the chicken pox virus causing shingles. Finally there could be a bug in the computer program you are using; this corresponds to a psychological disorder such as depression.

Evidently the treatment required to get the printer working again will vary considerably depending on what the cause is; some problems are simpler than others to solve, and if it turns out that the problem is complicated you may have to live with it or find a way around it. Of course, the analogy breaks down here, because if worse comes to worst you can always get a new computer or printer but you cannot get a new back or brain.

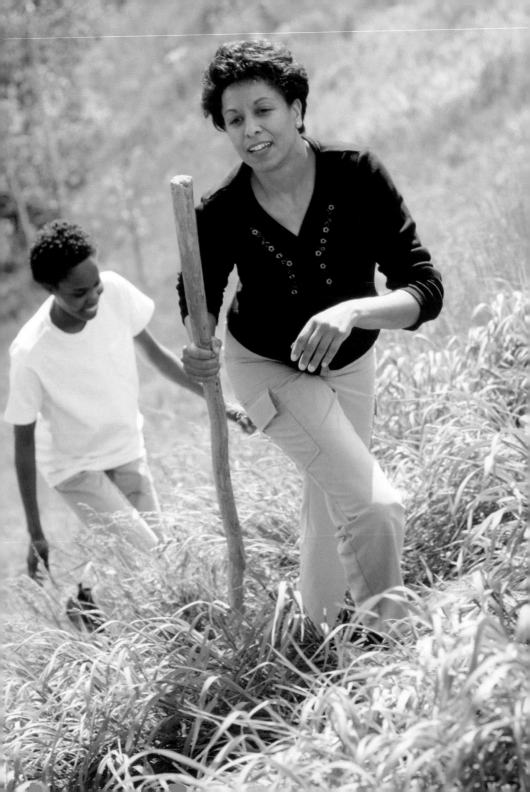

options
for a
healthy
back

What can you do to protect your back from pain, either if you have never had an attack or if you are seeking ways to avoid a recurrence of a long-standing problem? In this section we will outline some simple lifestyle changes that may help, ranging from better posture, stress-free housework, and choice of mattress to an improved driving position. We then concentrate on back exercises and the treatment of acute and chronic back pain before finally looking at different therapies and alternative solutions.

preventing
back pain

The boundary between the treatment and prevention of back pain is not fixed and some methods advised for prevention may also have a role in treatment. Many of the measures described here are used on an informal, self-help basis and are divided into changes you can adopt easily at home or in the office, or while driving and traveling. Some are more formal, such as the "back school" approach, in which anyone from office workers to nurses are taught proper posture.One of the other lessons taught in these schools is the right way to carry out various activities that people perform in their daily lives and at work. These are mostly measures that are sensible for everyone, whether or not they have had a previous attack of back pain.

Posture

Be aware of your posture when standing and sitting. Some people stand slouched, stomachs forward and with an exaggerated "hump" at the upper part of their back. This stance is more or less unavoidable in late pregnancy and for anyone who is seriously overweight, but even slim people sometimes slouch. It results in excessive strain in the lumbar and upper thoracic regions and is an important cause of backaches, especially in younger people; older people tend to have adapted to their "abnormal" posture and are unable to change it.

If you are below middle age with a slouch,you should make a conscious effort to correct it, although it is important not to go too far the other way. The military "correct position of attention," with a supererect spine, shoulders braced back, and an exaggerated hollow in the lumbar region, is also undesirable, causing strain on the lumbar spine and aching in the neck and shoulders.

How should you stand? The problem with trying to correct postural faults yourself is that your standing position is so natural to you that any alteration in it, even to a posture that is anatomically "better," is bound to seem strange at first. Indeed, you may well not be able to improve your posture unaided. If so, you might benefit from advice from a physiotherapist, osteopath (p. 14), or Alexander Technique teacher (pp. 123–124). As a general rule for life you should avoid extreme positions or extreme stress for long periods, which means for more than an

Back schools are used by companies to teach employees how to avoid the types of injury often incurred through long periods of office work. Here a back chair is being demonstrated.

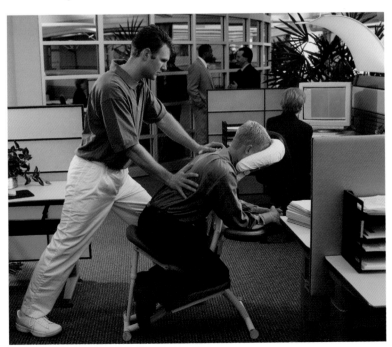

hour at a time. Discover by experiment what suits you best. Be prepared to try things out, while keeping in mind the basic structure of the back and how it functions (see "The Structure of the Back" pp. 14–23).

How should you sit? Many chairs, especially so-called "easy chairs," appear to have been deliberately designed to encourage those who sit in them to adopt a bad posture. You are more or less forced to slouch, with curved spine and head sticking forward like a pecking chicken. To correct this as far as possible, place a cushion behind your lumbar spine and bring your head back until it is in line with your spine. If you are watching television you may need to change the height of the set. For reading, your book should be propped up at an angle rather than lying flat so that you do not have to look down at it.

Choosing a chair Check to see how far it permits the adoption of a functionally correct posture. Some back sufferers derive benefit from a radically different type of chair, in which you half-sit, half-kneel; the seat is angled slightly forward and part of the body weight is taken by a second support beneath the knees. These "back chairs," as they are called, tend to be rather expensive but they are worth considering for anyone whose work or leisure involves much sitting. If they are used for a long time, however, you may get sore knees.

When you don't need to sit upright, a fairly radical option is a zero-gravity chair. These are based on chairs originally designed for astronauts in space. A wide variety of other chairs is now available, including massage chairs, orthopedic chairs, and ergonomic chairs. Obviously the best test of these is to try them out for yourself, and they can be expensive. A simpler option for sitting at home is to place a footstool in front of your favorite sofa or armchair. Alternatively, many sofas and armchairs are now made with footrests that flip out from underneath. This should help relieve strain placed on the lumbar region when sitting. No matter what chair you use, at home or at work, it is always advisable to get up regularly and walk around.

Sleep

Few subjects have attracted more mythology than the right choice of bed for back sufferers. The widespread belief that "the firmer the better" is misleading; in fact, too firm a bed can be almost as bad as one that sags. So-called "orthopedic" mattresses may be no better, or even worse, than ordinary ones costing a fraction of the price.

Choosing a bed To a considerable extent the choice of a suitable bed and mattress has to be a matter of trial and error, but unfortunately just lying for a few minutes on a bed in a store showroom is not really an adequate test; there is no substitute for sleeping on a bed for several nights to find out whether it really suits you. The ideal is to find a mattress that keeps your spine in as neutral a position as possible: that is, when you are lying on your side your spine should be more or less in a straight line. If your hips or shoulders are wide this position may be better achieved on a fairly soft mattress than on a harder one. However, the base of the bed, as opposed to the mattress, should not be excessively soft.

When lying in bed, try to get your spine as straight as possible by choosing an appropriate number of pillows and a suitable mattress, neither too firm nor too soft.

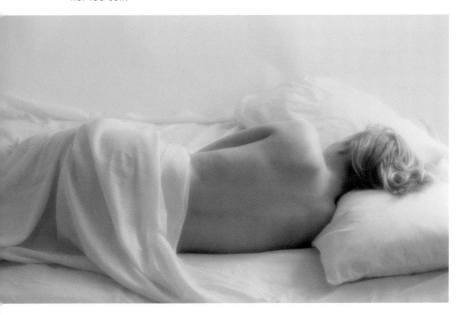

Pillows The number of pillows is, like the mattress, a question of individual choice, but use the same guideline: keep the spine more or less horizontal. Obviously the consistency of the pillows is important; avoid the springy kind filled with a compound that does not compress much since this will not mold itself to your contours. For most people two fairly soft pillows are probably best, and should be replaced when they have lost most of their bulk. Whether you use one or two pillows, tuck them well under your neck, rather than placing the support at your head and leaving a gap at your neck. Special horseshoe-shaped pillows are available to provide this kind of support though you can achieve the same effect with a rolled-up towel. There are now many companies in the United States offering orthopedic, chiropractic, or water pillows – you can find them on the Internet.

If you consistently wake up in the morning with a stiff neck, it is well worth considering whether your neck posture during the night is satisfactory.

Reading in bed This is difficult without straining your neck, and back. If you lie with your head propped up on pillows you are liable to give yourself neck pain, while if you sit upright with your legs in front of you there will probably be some strain on your lumbar spine. It may be better to avoid reading in bed altogether (and this practice is generally discouraged anyway if you suffer from insomnia). If you must read, however, at least change your position frequently, perhaps alternating between sitting with three pillows behind your back and lying on your side with a pillow under your lumbar spine to keep your back horizontal.

Sex

If you or your partner suffers from neck or back pain you will probably find that sex becomes difficult and becomes less frequent or even nonexistent, either because it is painful or because you fear that it may be harmful. This problem is seldom much talked about, perhaps because either patients or their therapists are embarrassed. This is a pity because it is generally unnecessary to discontinue sexual relations when you have a back problem and good sex will have a therapeutic effect in itself.

Fear of pain or injury Sexual difficulties in back pain sufferers can arise in two main ways. One is psychological. If you are anxious, depressed, or simply in pain, you are unlikely to be able to function sexually in a normal way. Fear of pain or injury may well be enough in itself to inhibit a sexual response. If so, try discussing it frankly with your partner. If you cannot resolve it in this way, ask for help from your doctor, a licensed counselor or psychotherapist, or a mental health clinic. It is often possible to find a way of solving problems of this kind. If fear of damage to your spine is what inhibits you, cognitive behavioral therapy of the kind discussed in "Treating Chronic Back Pain" (p.103) should enable you to discover that the fear may not be based on reality.

The other main source of difficulty, which may overlap with the psychological factors, is finding a comfortable position for sex. There is no single answer to this, so experiment and find what works best for you and your partner. A strategically placed pillow or towel will often make this easier. A good position is often for both partners to lie on their sides in an S-shape, but sometimes sitting may be easier than lying down; there are no rules. If you experience back pain during intercourse, tell your partner at once and suggest you change your positions.

As with the psychological difficulties, you should seek professional help if you

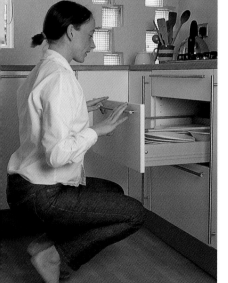

cannot solve things on your own. Find a health professional who is happy to discuss these matters with you; many are.

Movement

In carrying out the everyday activities of living it is important to strike a balance between reasonable care for one's back and excessive caution. As we will see in the discussion of chronic back pain, fear of movement (see "Treating Chronic Back Pain", p.104) is often part of a vicious circle of pain avoidance and loss of function.

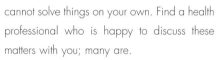

When reaching for a low object, squat rather than stoop; bend your knees rather than your back.

Fear If you find yourself in the situation of being unable to do many things for fear of damaging your back you should probably consider trying to find a center offering the kind of multidisciplinary approach described in "Treating Chronic Back Pain" (pp. 102–105). Nevertheless, it is sensible to know which kinds of movements are best avoided and how to perform daily tasks in a way that minimizes the risk of harm.

Bending and twisting The worst kind of movement is probably bending forward and twisting the back at the same time, since this imposes stress on the disks at the moment when they are most vulnerable. Almost as risky is lifting a weight with arms outstretched. This exerts a strong leverage on the spine that has to be counteracted by strong contraction of the spinal muscles. Avoiding the need to do these things is largely a matter of thought and anticipation, but certain kinds of activity warrant particular attention. If you suffer from recurrent or chronic back pain you need to think about all the things you do habitually at home and at work, analyse them, and modify them as necessary.

At the same time, don't concentrate exclusively on the mechanics of lifting. These are important, but so is the smoothness and fluidity with which any movement is performed. If you watch a cat you see a wonderful demonstration of how to move; your aim should be to make all your movements, especially those related to lifting, as catlike as possible.

Footwear

It has been said for many years that wearing high heels is likely to cause back problems because the natural balance of the body is upset. Intuitively it seems reasonable that this would be the case, since the high heels tilt the pelvis and lower back forward and this might place a strain on the muscles and ligaments. However, the heel height issue is really part of a wider question, concerning the relation between footwear and back pain, which is being studied by podiatrists (foot specialists). It is thought that excessive pronation (inward rotation) of the foot occurs, often because the big toe is unduly stiff. This excessive twisting causes other joints to move abnormally to compensate, and when these movements are repeated millions of times a year, problems with the spine may result. When this is thought to be the case, patients are given inserts to place in their shoes, called orthotic

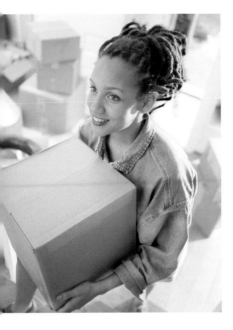

When lifting, keep the load as close to your body as possible to reduce the mechanical strain on your spine.

devices. These must be designed individually for each patient.

This work is still at an early stage and it is certainly not the case that alterations in foot function are involved in all, or even many, back problems. Nevertheless, this possibility may be worth considering, especially if you know that you have any abnormality in your feet, especially a stiff big toe. And if you are considering taking up any form of sport or regular walking you should certainly take advice about your choice of footwear

On the move

A handbag or shoulder bag, especially if it is heavy, can place undue strain on the neck and shoulder muscles as well as on the spine itself. If it is essential to carry a load in this way you should change the side frequently to even out the strain.

Using a backpack may also give rise to symptoms when you go on vacation. It is worth paying extra to get a backpack that has a good frame, which will spread the load.

If you are a cyclist it is better to carry loads in a saddlebag or basket rather than in a backpack; let the bicycle take the strain!

Lifting

Lifting is probably the single activity that causes most anxiety. The general aim should be to lift with the weight as close to you as possible and with your spine as straight (vertical) as possible. Stooping to lift is therefore undesirable. You should always have a secure foothold. Avoid stooping, especially with straight or nearly straight knees; your hips should always be lower than your head. Lifting should be done smoothly, without snatching or jerking, and if you need to turn with the weight you should do so by swiveling your feet instead of twisting your back. When you put the article down you should repeat the same movement that you made when picking it up: once again avoid stooping; squat instead. Don't hold even light articles at arms' length; always bring them in close to your body to minimize the load on your spine.

Avoid stooping If you are lifting wet clothes out of a washing machine, train yourself to squat beside the machine and bend your knees rather than your back. Ironing is best done sitting down, to avoid the strain caused by leaning forward with the weight of the iron in your hand. Lifting small children, especially at bath-time, needs care. Again, squat rather than stoop. When the children are still quite small it is better to bathe them in a tub placed on a table rather than to lean into an adult-sized bath.

Heavy lifting Before moving heavy items such as furniture, work out the best way to do it. If possible, heavy articles should be maneuvred onto low trolleys, but if this cannot be done, at least avoid pushing them from their upper part, which is more difficult. Usually it is better to sit on the floor and push them with your feet at the lowest part, ideally with your back braced against a wall.

Shopping Carry loads from the store divided equally into two, one part in each hand. This evens the strain on your spine. You could use a shopping basket but most of these are poorly designed and may themselves cause backstrain. When shopping by car in a supermarket avoid overfilling the individual bags; better to have many lighter bags rather than a few heavy ones. Be careful when loading heavy items into the trunk and taking them out — a trunk with a low ledge will make this easier.

In the home

The kitchen sink should be set at a comfortable height, neither too high nor too low. If it is too high you will have to lift things out at arms' length. Of course, it is difficult to alter the height of a sink but if necessary you can stand on something stable. If it is too low you could place an inverted bowl in the sink or put a board across it.

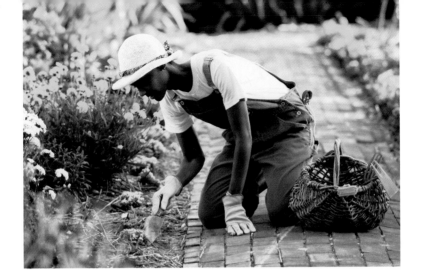

Weeding is not usually heavy work, but you should kneel rather than stoop. This gardener should be using a kneeling mat to protect the knees.

When dusting or polishing you should try to avoid making repeated movements with one arm. Change hands frequently to ease the strain on your back. Similarly, when using a vacuum cleaner, especially a heavy one, change hands frequently and walk along with it instead of pushing it a long way away from your body.

Making beds may involve shaking heavy blankets or turning mattresses. Shaking blankets out of the window places great strain on the lower back. Try to find help with these things instead of doing them on your own.

Hair washing, making up, and shaving Try to avoid leaning forward across a sink to peer at yourself in a mirror. This places a lot of strain on your lower back and neck. Whenever possible, sit rather than stand, or have a mirror mounted on an arm so that you don't need to lean over.

Dressing Putting on socks, panty hose, and shoes is difficult if your back is stiff or painful. Try to avoid bending over or standing on one leg; sit down on a bed or a chair instead. A long-handled shoehorn will help with tight shoes. Shoelaces should be tied by placing your foot on a chair and leaning forward against your knee so that your trunk is supported. (Incidentally, this is also the posture recommended as an exercise for stretching the *psoas* muscle – see Exercise 12, p. 92.)

In the garden

Many gardening tasks can bring on back symptoms in those at risk. Digging involves lifting, usually with a bent back. Gardening "claws" are now widely available. These require a twisting action from the user in order to spiral the claws through the earth, and require less physical effort than the traditional shovel. Another option, initially proposed for elderly or wheelchair-bound gardeners, but suitable for anyone with back problems, is to have raised flowerbeds. These are beds built into structures usually about a foot or two high, with paths around them, which can be worked on comfortably from a chair, or even if kneeling, means the gardener can stay virtually upright instead of bending and stooping.

Pushing a lawn mower requires the gardener to exert a good deal of force while leaning forward. If you must do these things yourself, at least stop and rest frequently. Weeding, although not heavy work, may mean lots of bending over, so kneel on a rubberized mat.

The standard design of wheelbarrow seems to be especially adapted to place strain on the back. Avoid overloading the wheelbarrow; it is better to make more trips with lighter loads.

Clearing snow is potentially dangerous for anyone unused to hard exertion, especially the middle-aged and elderly. This is not only because of the strain on the back, but because the unaccustomed exertion may be risky for the heart, especially in the cold air that can affect blood flow in the heart muscle. It may be wiser to leave the snow to melt or find someone else to do the work.

DIY

Many do-it-yourself activities can be difficult if you have back or neck problems. The precautions about heavy lifting apply. Another area of concern is any kind of work that requires looking up for long periods. Putting up curtains, fixing lights, and especially painting ceilings, are particularly hazardous for people with spondylosis (pp. 31–32) in the neck. It is common for patients to say that after doing these things for a few hours they have pain in their head, neck, shoulders, or arms for several days or even longer.

There is an important artery called the vertebrobasilar artery that supplies the lower part of the brain and travels up the spine through special apertures in the transverse processes of the cervical vertebrae. If your cervical spine is suffering from "wear-and-tear" changes, looking up or sideways for long periods can compress this artery. This should be avoided since it could make you faint. If looking upward makes you dizzy, standing on a ladder while painting a ceiling, for instance, can be dangerous. If you do paint the ceiling or something of that kind, it is a good idea to take regular breaks, kneel on all fours, and let the head hang down for a few minutes.

At work

Employers are increasingly aware of the need to prevent back injuries to their employees. Manual laborers and nurses, or anyone involved in heavy lifting, are particularly at risk. But even office work has its hazards; heavy files may need to be lifted and sitting at a desk for long periods is bad for the back, which needs to be kept mobile if it is to remain healthy. The introduction of back schools in some work settings (see p.71), is one solution to the problem.

Good working practice In order to help yourself at work you should always remember the advice about lifting: squat rather than bend, keep the object you are lifting close to your body, and avoid twisting your back while carrying a weight. If you work at a keyboard, think about your posture, using the same criteria as were discussed earlier in relation to "How should you sit?" (see p. 60). If your work involves spending long stretches of time on the phone, use a hands-free set or headset. If you do a lot of copying, don't lay the material flat on the desk; instead, prop it up in front of you so that you do not need to keep looking down. Slouching and poking your head forward are bad; you should aim for an upright but not supererect posture.

If you use a monitor you should give some thought to its positioning. Many people seem to put it on top of their computer, but this often makes it necessary for them to keep looking upward, which can place a strain on the neck. It may be better to have the screen lower than this so that you are looking horizontally or slightly downward.

Much pain in the neck and shoulders arises because the desk is too high. It should be positioned so that your arms are roughly parallel to the floor. Don't sit too near your desk or too far away. If you have difficulty in achieving the right position, use an adjustable chair.

Keep moving No matter how good your posture may be, you should not try to maintain it continuously for long periods. Every 20 to 30 minutes, therefore, you should move around, look away from your work, and perhaps stand up for a minute. Shrugging the shoulders often gives relief from neck and shoulder stiffness; also, stretch your fingers and perform simple neck exercises of the kind described in "Exercises for Your Back" (pp. 87–88). It is important not to wait for pain to develop; you should make the movements regularly to prevent the symptoms rather than to cure them. If necessary, keep a watch beside your desk to remind you to take breaks at regular intervals.

Take care with your posture when driving, by ensuring that your seat is a comfortable distance from the foot pedals, and is in an adequately upright position. Make sure the headrest is high enough in case of a rear impact that could cause whiplash injury. NOTE: your headrest should be higher than shown here!

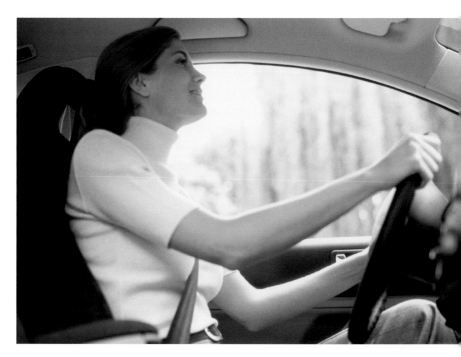

Back schools

Back schools originated in Sweden in the 1980s. In four sessions of 45 minutes, participants were taught about the anatomy and function of the back and about the role of mechanical stress in causing back pain. They also received advice about exercises to improve their back and were encouraged to adopt a more active lifestyle. Back schools were set up by companies to try to improve the health of their employees. Today the teaching seems to vary widely; some take a more intensive approach than others. In one case, for example, nurses with a history of back pain followed a five-week program in a back clinic for eight hours a day; at least four hours a day was spent doing exercises and the nurses also received ergonomic education, individual physiotherapy, and behavioral therapy. Intensive programs of this kind seem to give the best results, with a period of between three and five weeks in a specialized center.

Driving

Traveling by car seems to cause more problems to back sufferers than almost anything else. Even people who normally do not have back symptoms often find that they get back pain when driving. There are several possible reasons for this.

The problem with car seats The most obvious reason for back pain when driving is posture. Both drivers and passengers, but especially drivers, are fixed in one position for long periods. Few cars seem to have seats that are ergonomically designed to give the right support for the back, and, in any case, it would be difficult to have seats that were right for everyone. There are so many variations in height, weight, and build that the seating must always be something of a compromise. Things are nevertheless improving; many cars have fully adjustable seats to give better lumbar support. You should consider these things carefully when choosing a new car, but unfortunately, a few minutes spent sitting in a car, or even going for a short test drive, are not usually enough to let you judge the long-term suitability of a car for your back. You really need to spend at least several hours in the car, but this is seldom possible unless you happen to have a friend who owns a similar car. It is sometimes possible to improve a less than ideal seat by means of a cushion or a back support.

Driving position It is not only the characteristics of the seat that matter; so do the height and angle of the steering wheel, which can sometimes be adjusted. The pedal positions are fixed, however, and these matter, too. The seat should be the correct distance from the steering wheel, which you should check regularly if you share a car. A heavy clutch can cause back pain in some people, especially in town driving where many gear changes are required. There is a strong case for choosing automatic transmission if frequent gear changes aggravate your back pain.

Neck, shoulder, and arm stiffness A common complaint when driving is of pain and stiffness in the neck, shoulders, and arms – hardly surprising since driving for long periods, especially on freeways, keeps you more or less motionless. So turn your head frequently, relax your grip on the steering wheel, and shrug your shoulders whenever the traffic comes to a halt. A lower- back pillow may also be helpful. On the freeway, stop at service stations at least every hour, and get out of the car and walk around. This not only helps your back but reduces sleepiness.

Adjust headrests The height of the headrests should be high enough to reach the back of the head. Set too low they may make matters worse in the event of a collision, by providing a pivot around which the neck can be stretched, thus increasing the chance of a whiplash injury (see pp. 33–34).

Avoid tension Not all the pain that drivers experience is due to faulty posture, badly designed seating, or immobility. Psychological factors are also involved. Psychological tension makes us clench our muscles, especially those of the neck, shoulders, and face, and causes us to grip the steering wheel too tightly. Indeed, the tone (see p. 20) of every muscle may be increased. Driving in modern traffic conditions is inevitably stressful, but making a conscious decision to cultivate as detached an attitude as possible to annoying incidents that inevitably occur helps to counteract this. Meditation and similar techniques can help.

Loading the car Take care when putting heavy items into the trunk or taking them out. Try to choose a car that does not have a high ledge over which things have to be lifted, and divide the load into several small items.

Several aspects of car travel are liable to produce twisting movements of the spine. And remember, if your neck is stiff you may find reversing difficult, which is a real problem, especially in parking. Be careful about turning to lift things out of the backseat. When getting into or out of the car, train yourself to do so by swiveling your whole body around on your buttocks rather than twisting your spine.

Car maintenance Changing a tire is potentially hazardous. First, you have to undo the lug nuts, which may be tight. Don't pull on the wheel rim with bent back, but use your weight by stepping on the arm of the rim. (Keep the lug nuts greased and ask the garage not to tighten the nuts excessively.) Having loosened the nuts, you have to lift the spare tire out of the trunk and replace it with the punctured tire. Tires are heavy, so be careful. In fact, if you are a back sufferer it is probably wise to join a roadside rescue organization and avoid the need to change tires altogether.

If you are an amateur car mechanic you will probably spend a lot of time peering into the depths of your car engine. This can put a lot of strain on your lower back. You may need to curtail your car maintenance or at least divide up the tasks so as to avoid doing too much in a day or a weekend. Also, try to rest one foot on the bumper, or place a support for your foot on the ground near the car.

PREVENTING OSTEOPOROSIS

Young people should take plenty of exercise and build up their calcium stores throughout life by including vitamin D and calcium-rich food such as dairy products in their diet. Green-leaf vegetables and nuts are an alternative source of calcium for people wishing to avoid dairy products. People at risk of osteoporosis, such as menopausal women, can have bone density estimations to assess the condition of their bones. Hormone replacement is proven to improve bone density (though there is no evidence yet that it reduces the rate of fractures) and is usually advised for women who have an early menopause. There are also drugs, such as calcitonin (a hormone) that can reduce osteoporosis. Weight-bearing exercise is also helpful.

Air travel

Packing for a long trip is stressful enough without having to worry about whether you can carry your loaded suitcases around the airport without straining tender back muscles.

Organize your luggage As with shopping, it is best to divide the luggage you need to carry into several smaller pieces rather than pack all your belongings into one large case. Pulling a suitcase with wheels obviously makes things easier but will involve twisting the back, so you should swap it from arm to arm. Lifting the suitcase or cases onto the conveyer belt at the checkout desk can be difficult. Ask for help; don't be tempted to risk it.

Once your luggage is checked in you should have only one, fairly light, piece of hand luggage left to cope with, but if you visit the duty-free shop you may acquire some surprisingly heavy items, so be careful.

Green-leaf vegetables such as cabbage, broccoli, and brussel sprouts provide essential vitamins and minerals that are needed for healthy bones and joints.

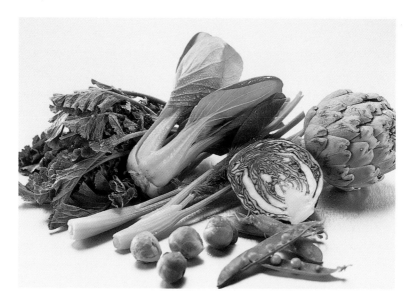

Wheelchair Severe chronic back pain sufferers should consider circumventing all these problems by asking in advance for a wheelchair at both departure and destination. As an added bonus you will probably go through the formalities at the airport more quickly than will your more mobile fellow passengers.

On the plane If the seat numbers are allocated in advance you should ask for a place where there is more than the usual leg room. Accommodations are usually cramped, especially on charter flights. If you are in the air for many hours you should get out of your seat and move around from time to time, at least once an hour. This will not only reduce the strain on your back but help to prevent the possibility of a deep vein thrombosis. If your seat forces you into a poor posture, ask the cabin attendant for a cushion to place behind the small of your back. If you need to sleep or rest, and do not have a full-reclining seat, travel pillows can be very helpful. These are inflatable horseshoe-shaped pillows that fit neatly around your neck and will support the weight of your head if you lean it to one side, thus relieving the strain on the neck.

Nutrition

The nutritional aspect of preventing back pain should not be forgotten. Eating large quantities of "junk food" will tend to result in being overweight, which is harmful in itself. Excess fat places more strain on your back, especially if the fat is mainly located in the abdomen or breasts where it exerts greater leverage on the spine. However, it is not helpful to become too preoccupied with your weight; relatively modest degrees of overweight will not affect back pain significantly. Losing weight and keeping it off is notoriously difficult; probably the best hope of doing so is to join one of the self-help groups that exist for the purpose.

Junk food is likely to be deficient in vitamins and trace elements such as zinc and magnesium that are necessary for maintenance of the tissues. Vitamins C and D are particularly important: healing after injury and the formation of strong scars depends on vitamin C, and vitamin D is needed for maintaining strong bones. However, this does not mean that you have to take nutritional supplements; these should be unnecessary provided your diet contains plenty of fresh fruit and vegetables as well as a wide variety of other foods. The kind of advice that is given to everyone to prevent heart disease will also help to maintain the health of the back.

exercises
for your **back**

There are two aspects to exercise in relation to back pain: first, exercise in general, and second, exercises for specific types of back pain. However, although there is strong evidence to suggest that general exercise is good for the back, the value of specific back exercises is uncertain. And while exercise in moderation is highly desirable, some forms, if care is not taken, can do more harm than good.

The health of the back should not be thought of in isolation but as part of general health, and it is certainly always desirable to maintain a basic level of fitness. The main kind of fitness that is relevant here is cardiovascular — the heart, lungs, and circulation. There is no need to try to become an Olympic athlete. Even modest levels of fitness and activity will benefit not only your general health, including your back, but will help control weight — an ever-increasing problem for many people. Our largely sedentary lifestyle is one of the main factors contributing to obesity, heart attacks, hypertension, and diabetes.

So far as the back is concerned, weight-bearing exercise helps to combat osteoporosis (see p.39) although not all forms of exercise are equally effective. In short, the exercise should stress the bone that is to be protected. For example, we know that running and jumping stress the hips and this helps to prevent hip fractures, but the role of exercise in preventing vertebral fractures is less clear.

The health of the disks depends in part on movement, and exercise is relevant here as well. So taking the spine, and particularly the neck, regularly through its full range of pain-free movement is a good thing.

Exercise also has important psychological benefits. As we saw in "Symptoms and Their Causes" (pp. 25, 34, 35, 45–46) earlier, depression is an important factor in chronic back pain. Exercise has repeatedly been shown to be effective in relieving depression and altering mood, and it is therefore likely to help those back sufferers whose condition is, in part, due to their depression.

Exercise throughout life

The benefits of exercise apply regardless of age. Even people in their '80s and '90s can respond to exercise programs and increase their strength, and exercises for this age group have been shown to reduce the incidence of falls. However, it is only sensible to take your general state of health and fitness, or unfitness, into account. It would be foolish to rush into vigorous exercise without preparation. And, if you are over 40, and you suffer from high blood pressure, diabetes, or any long-term disease of the heart or lungs, or you are seriously overweight, you should consult your doctor before attempting any sort of vigorous exercise. Walking, on the other hand, is suitable for almost everyone.

If an exercise program is to be successful it has to be reasonably pleasant and cause minimal disruption to your normal lifestyle, otherwise you will be unlikely to keep it up. Continuity is important, since fitness is lost quite rapidly once exercise ceases. The best forms of exercise are those that involve repeated movement of large muscle groups (those in the back and legs). These include walking, jogging and running, swimming, cycling, and dancing.

Some games, such as golf and tennis, can also be beneficial, but both of these may aggravate back problems because they tend to involve twisting movements. Squash is potentially dangerous for middle-aged people who are not used to it. It requires sudden bursts of exertion that may be a risk to the heart, and the strong competitive element raises blood pressure.

Whatever form of exercise you choose, apart from walking, you should warm up gradually and also slow down gradually. To switch abruptly from rest to vigorous exertion is undesirable even for young, fit people and can be fatal for the middle-aged and elderly. It can strain unprepared muscles, ligaments, and joints. Many books and articles advise a program of stretching before exercise, but recent research questions that it makes a difference.

Walking

This is the simplest, and for many people the best, form of exercise. It need not be very demanding. As little as 20 minutes' fairly brisk walking three or four times a week is enough to provide a worthwhile degree of fitness. There is no need to buy special clothing and walking can simply mean going to the store or to work on foot. Walk whenever possible instead of driving. There are, however, one or two things to look out for if you suffer with your back.

Precautions Avoid carrying even a light load such as a camera or field glasses around your neck, which can strain it. Use a belt so that the weight is carried by your pelvis. Walking a dog may seem a good way to encourage you to go out even when the weather is not inviting, but the pull of a large dog on a lead can cause a surprising amount of back pain. So, make sure that your dog is trained to walk on its lead without pulling. Grandparents who take care of a toddler for a week or two may find the hand tugging they get, or pushing a stroller, sets off an attack of back pain.

As with any form of unaccustomed exercise, you should start off gradually, walking perhaps for 10 minutes a day initially and increasing the distance as fitness improves. If walking brings on back pain you should consult a physiotherapist or osteopath. It could also be worth seeing a podiatrist if you suspect your footwear is to blame.

Running and jogging

There is no agreed definition of jogging; it really seems to be the same as running rather slowly. Running is more demanding than walking and produces the same amount of fitness in a shorter time, but it is not suitable for everyone, either because of age or health problems or simply because it's not enjoyable. It is certainly possible to achieve the same effects just by walking if you are prepared to invest the time.

If you do take up running it is worth investing in a pair of good running shoes. If in doubt, seek advice from one of the specialized stores that sell equipment for runners. Also, pay attention to your posture when running. Many people carry their arms too high, which imposes a strain on their upper back and neck. If you find that

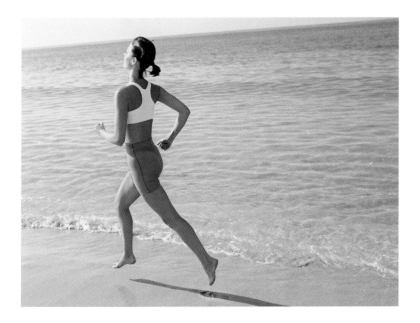

Running is a good form of exercise if you enjoy it, but pay attention to your posture; do not carry your arms too high or hunch your shoulders.

you suffer from neckaches or backaches after running, this is a sign that something is wrong with your technique; running clubs will offer expert advice.

Swimming

This is often recommended to back sufferers, and with good reason. Swimming uses arm and leg movements that are sometimes recommended for back pain, and because the body and limbs are supported by the water there is less strain on the joints and ligaments than when walking or running. However, since it is weight-bearing exercise that tends to counteract osteoporosis, swimming does not help, but it does have some effect in reducing body fat.

The choice of stroke is important for back sufferers. The front crawl is good provided you breathe on both sides instead of one, but not everyone is able to use this stroke effectively. The breaststroke is also good provided you can do it properly. This means keeping your body in more or less a straight line, which requires

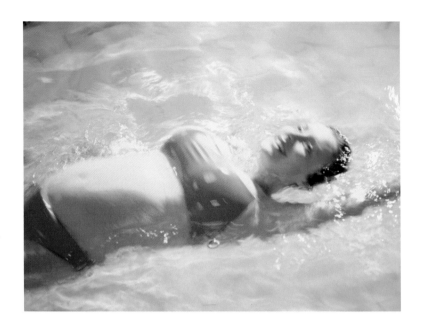

The backstroke may be better for your neck than swimming on your front because your head is supported by the water.

exhaling while your mouth is underwater and raising your head only to inhale as you sweep your arms around and back. If you swim with your head out of the water all the time this will impose an undesirable strain on your neck and back muscles. An alternative to the breaststroke is the backstroke, which may indeed be the best position so far as your back is concerned.

Even if you cannot swim at all, this does not mean that the pool has nothing to offer you. You may derive benefit simply from splashing around vigorously against the resistance of the water in the shallow end.

Cycling

Cycling has many potential advantages for back pain sufferers. As a weight-bearing exercise it falls between walking or running on the one hand and swimming on the other; the body is partly supported by the saddle, which can suit people with arthritis of their knees or other leg problems. At least one study has found that

CHOOSING A BIKE

Choose your bicycle carefully. It is unwise to buy something by mail order; go to a specialized bicycle dealer and explain your requirements. Most bicycles sold these days are of the semi-upright type and this is generally suitable for back pain patients. There are many different designs, some of which have shock absorbers and shock-absorbent seats. These are primarily intended for riding on rough ground but they can be advantageous for back pain sufferers because they cushion road bumps too. The extra cost is probably worth it.

Whatever type of bicycle you choose, it is essential to make sure that it is the right size. Too small and you will be hunched up, while if it is too large you will have to reach forward too far to grasp the handlebars. Both positions are common causes of backache and neckache. Even if the size is right the bicycle must be correctly adjusted for you. Important points to check are the height of the handlebars and saddle. If you are getting neck pain it may be that the handlebars are set too low, causing you to look up; while if the saddle is set too high you will rock your pelvis from side to side as you pedal. Once again, advice from a knowledgeable dealer or from a cycling club will help.

patients with lung diseases (chronic bronchitis and emphysema) can get around better on a bicycle than on foot because they tend to lean forward more so the lines of stress on their spine tend to be different. Patients suffering from narrowing of the lumbar spinal canal (spinal stenosis) who find walking is painful can often find cycling more comfortable, again because it forces them to lean forward.

Radical alternative An alternative to the conventional bicycle is a recumbent type. As the name implies, you sit semihorizontally with your back supported by a rest. This is not a machine that a newcomer to cycling would be likely to consider, but it does have possibilities for enthusiasts who may have given up their sport because of back pain. Some have found that such a bike is better for their backs

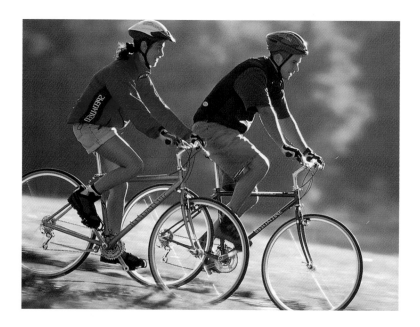

Cycling is a very good form of exercise but it is important that your bicycle is the right size and that the saddle is adjusted to the correct height for you.

than the ordinary kind; others say that pushing against the pedals is rather like pressing a heavy clutch in a car, and this makes their pain worse.

Riding a stationary cycle is certainly a valid way of maintaining fitness but can be boring. It also makes you very hot while real cycling creates a cooling breeze. However, it does have two merits: it is not affected by the weather and it avoids the risks of riding on the road. To overcome the monotony of fixed cycling, many fitness centers offer classes in what they term "spinning." This is a studio full of fixed bicycles, sometimes with a large screen projecting a moving scenic road route. An instructor will then take you on a virtual cycle ride, including hills, flat stretches, and fast and slow phases.

Dancing

Dancing appeals to many people and it can be excellent exercise. You can choose the level of exertion according to taste, and the movements involved are often of the kind likely to help osteoporosis and the general condition of the spine. If you do experience back pain after dancing, you need to modify, or moderate your movements. Some forms of Latin American dancing, such as salsa and lambada, which involve lots of pelvic movement, back arching, and sudden backward drops, can exert high amounts of strain on the lumbar region. Some "break dancers," who use violent head movements, have suffered serious injuries to their necks, sometimes leading to paralysis from spinal artery thrombosis.

If you do take up any form of dancing, it is essential to take classes with a qualified instructor, at the right level for you. You should also inform the dance teacher of any previous or current back problems so that they can advise you on which moves might be particularly beneficial, and which ones you may need to avoid.

Postural exercise disciplines

Exercise regimes such as yoga and Pilates have become hugely popular recently, and appeal to people who may also want a spiritual component to their physical exercise. This is by no means essential however, and these disciplines are widely promoted for their benefits to posture, flexibility, and muscle tone. Please see "Physical Therapies" pp. 123–125 for more detailed information about these therapies.

THEORETICAL BENEFITS OF EXERCISE

There is not much agreement about how exercises are supposed to work or what they are expected to achieve. Theories that have been put forward include

- *relieving pressure on nerve roots*
- *shifting nuclear material away from a bulging disk*
- *increasing the blood levels of naturally occurring pain-relieving substances called endorphins*
- *strengthening weak muscles*
- *decreasing mechanical stress*
- *stabilizing excessively mobile spinal segments*
- *improving posture and mobility*
- *increasing the input of pain-blocking nerve impulses in the spinal cord*

It is unlikely that all of these can be correct, but they do all make good sense.

Exercise balls

These large vinyl balls have been used by physical therapists for years to treat orthopedic disorders, but are now hugely popular with mainstream fitness instructors, and people can be seen using them in any health club or fitness center. They are affordable and can be bought for use at home. Many gyms offer classes in how to exercise with them, and books are also available.

The virtue of these balls is that they support the arch of the back and bear your weight while you exercise, and they can work several muscle groups deeply at the same time. They can help improve muscle tone and flexibility, and strengthen the abdominals and lower back.

Back exercises

Many popular books on the back place great emphasis on the use of specific exercises for the relief and prevention of back pain. It is easy to understand their appeal. Sufferers can perform these exercises without supervision, they are pretty safe, and if they work they are a welcome alternative to more drastic treatments such as surgery. Unfortunately there is not a great deal of evidence for the effectiveness of exercises of this kind. Nor is there yet conclusive evidence as to which kinds of exercise are most likely to help or which sufferers are best suited therefore, and likely to benefit from them.

Exercise or physio? The latest research in *Spine* journal shows that exercise can be effective for back and neck pain. In chronic low-back pain the picture is more complicated. The benefit of exercises seems to be about as good as conventional physiotherapy, but no better. However, the main aim of treatment in chronic low-back pain is to restore patients to ordinary activity and allow them to go back to work, and exercises may be useful as part of a rehabilitation program.

In short, there is no point in doing exercises in acute back pain but in chronic back pain they will probably be beneficial. They might or might not help with pain but they could speed up your return to normal life. If, on the other hand, you find exercises a chore, don't think that by not doing them you are diminishing your chances of recovery. There is no information available at present to show that any one type of back exercise is better than another.

The pros and cons

If you are exercising unsupervized, the golden rule is: IF IT HURTS, DON'T DO IT!

You need to remember that exercises can do harm as well as good. Those described here should be safe but there are no absolutes in medicine and every

BEFORE AND AFTER EXERCISE

Certain practices before and after your exercise, will help you get the most out of your workout, and could also help prevent injury:
- *Wear appropriate clothing (i.e., that will not restrict movement) and footwear (see p. 64) that offers the necessary support and cushioning for the impact level of your exercise.*
- *Warm up (e.g., a few minutes of brisk walking or marching on the spot). This will get your heart pumping oxygen into your muscles, ready for exertion.*
- *Warm down after exercise (and wrap up warm) this is better for your muscles than a sudden cessation, and may help prevent sudden stiffness from setting in.*

individual is different. You should not do any exercises if you have a disease of the spine, such as rheumatoid arthritis or cancer, that might make it unstable. If you find that a particular exercise gives you pain afterward, don't persevere with it. A moderate amount of discomfort during an exercise is not necessarily a reason for stopping, but this should not be taken to excess. Never overstrain a joint.

Flexibility Many people do exercises to improve their flexibility, but some rather vague thinking exists about why this should be useful. Movement at joints, whether in the spine or elsewhere, can be limited by three things: ligaments, aging of the spine, and muscle tone.

Ligaments Adults' ligaments have reduced elasticity and ill-advised attempts to stretch them may do more harm than good. Movement limitation due to ligaments is not necessarily a bad thing because it stabilizes the joints; in fact, people who are "double-jointed," meaning they have abnormally lax ligaments that allow their joints to move through an unusually large range, may be more liable than others to suffer from osteoarthritis in later life.

Ageing of the Spine The second limitation is due to the fact that as our spines age, spikes of bone form at the margins of the vertebral bodies; these are called osteophytes. It is impossible to force the spinal joints to move against them and you should not force it.

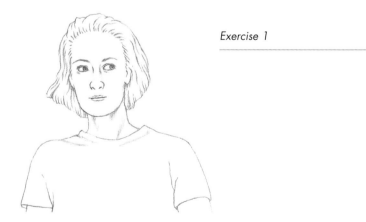

Exercise 1

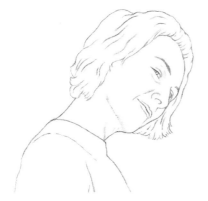

Muscle tone This is the only form of restriction that can be relaxed, and it is a good thing to do so by gently stretching the affected muscles. However, don't be tempted to do this by "bouncing." This increases the amount of tension because messages arrive from the spinal cord to tell the muscles to resist the movement.

As well as mobility, exercises can be designed to increase strength. There is no need to try to turn yourself into a Hercules, but if muscles have become weak as a result of immobility through pain or disuse, exercise should help to restore their health.

Neck exercises

The following exercises are designed to maintain or increase the range of neck movement and, in some cases, to build up strength. They can easily be performed in the home and do not require a lot of space. They should be safe (but refer to, "Exercise: pros and cons," above). If you are in any doubt, or experience any unusual sensations, stop and seek advice from a qualified therapist.

Exercise 1

To exercise the upper joints of your neck: sit in a chair and, placing your hands lightly in your lap, glide your head from side to side four or five times like a Balinese dancer; keep facing front but move your neck out to the side, back to center, and out to the other side. (If you are in doubt about what this entails, ask a physiotherapist.) This exercise should preferably be done first, before the nodding and turning exercises.

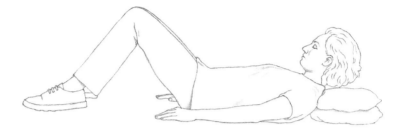

Exercise 2

Nodding exercise: sit on a firm chair without arms. With hands resting in your lap, look up at the ceiling and then down at the floor, meanwhile keeping your chin retracted; don't let your head poke forward. Repeat four or five times.

Exercise 3

Head-turning exercise: tilt your head downward at about 45 degrees, keeping your chin back. Turn your head to the left and right, alternately, as far as you comfortably can. Repeat four or five times in each direction.

Exercise 4

Some patients with **one-sided neck or shoulder pain** experience relief if the head is bent a few times toward the affected side. Pull your head down with your hand as far as you comfortably can, and hold it in place, without bending it either forward or backward, for about three seconds. Repeat once or twice. However, if this makes the pain worse, and especially if it begins to travel down the arm, don't persevere.

Exercise 5

To strengthen the muscles in the front of your neck: lie on your back on the floor with knees and hips bent, your feet flat on the floor, and your head supported on two pillows. Then raise your head smoothly, bringing your chin down toward your chest as far as possible (this also stretches the back of your neck). Repeat 10 to 20 times.

Exercise 6

Thoracic spine exercises

The main aim of exercises for this region is to maintain or improve mobility, especially in the upper part of the spine where many middle-aged and elderly people become stiff and immobile. An effective way of doing this is to stretch the muscles in the front of the chest (pectoral muscles).

Exercise 6

This helps **to relieve pain in the lower part of the neck** and also, perhaps unexpectedly, at the back of the neck and on top of the shoulders (what is sometimes called the yoke area): stand in a doorway with your arms outstretched, palms against each side of the doorway above your head like a letter "Y." Keeping your elbows straight, push your chest (not stomach) through the doorway as far as you can.

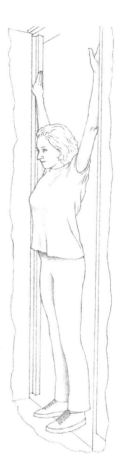

Exercise 8

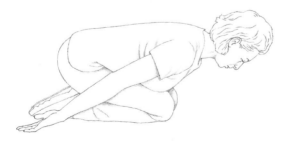

pelvis comes forward. At the same time tighten your buttock muscles. This exercise can be done standing as well as lying, and should be performed at intervals throughout the day.

Exercise 10

lie on the floor on your back and stretch downward with your left leg as far as you can, as if a string attached to the sole of you foot were being pulled toward the wall tilting your pelvis at the same time. Hold for a few seconds and then relax. Repeat the same exercise for your right leg. Repeat five to ten times each side.

Exercise 11

This exercise stretches the psoas muscle inside the abdomen: lie on the floor on your back and bend your left leg and hip until you can grasp your knee, and then pull your knee toward you with your hands. Hold for a few minutes and relax. Repeat with the right leg. Repeat five to ten times each side.

Exercise 12

This also stretches the psoas muscles: place your left foot on a chair with the leg straight and your right foot as far behind you as is comfortable. Keeping your right leg straight, bend your left knee slowly and lean forward until your chest rests on your left thigh (or comes as close to it as possible). Repeat with your right leg. Repeat 5 to 10 times. (Note that the RIGHT psoas muscle is stretched when the RIGHT foot is on the ground and vice versa.)

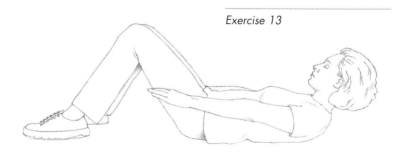

Exercise 13

Exercise 13

This exercise tones up your abdominal muscles: remember, increased strength and tone in your abdominal muscles will provide greater support for your spine.

Lie on your back on the floor with your knees and hips bent, and your feet flat on the floor. Smoothly, and without holding your breath, raise your head and the upper half of your body to an angle of about 20 degrees, or until you can see your insteps. Hold the posture for a few seconds; then lower them gently to the floor.

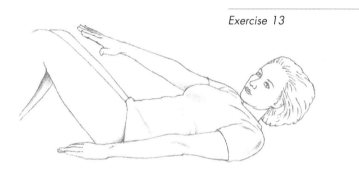

Exercise 13

You can also practice turning your trunk as you lift so as to bring each shoulder in turn toward your knees (see the second diagram for this exercise, above); this will exercise slightly different parts of the abdominal muscles. Repeat five to ten times.

Exercise 14

This exercise strengthens the big muscles of the back: lie face down on a strong table, with the edge of the table underneath your hips; use a folded towel as padding. Grip the top or sides of the table with your hands and then raise your legs and feet off the floor, bringing them as high in the air as you can. Lower your feet smoothly to the floor.

Repeat once or twice initially; build up gradually until you can do it five to ten times. If you find it difficult, don't force the movement but do as much as you comfortably can.

treating **acute** back pain

A first attack of back pain can be a frightening experience, especially if it comes on suddenly. You may find yourself unable to straighten up after bending over and the pain may be agonizing. So what should you do? The first thing is not to panic. Remember that most people recover from acute back pain in a few weeks and are able to resume all their normal activities. In the short term, however, you need to take measures to cope with the situation.

To rest or not?

At one time it was considered essential for anyone with acute back pain to go to bed, but nowadays the trend is very much in the opposite direction. Most studies show that recovery rates are the same whether people go to bed or remain active, and since there are definite risks, such as deep vein thrombosis (DVT) and osteoporosis, associated with remaining in bed for any length of time, it is generally thought best for patients to remain mobile and, if possible, at work. However, there is no need to take this advice to an extreme; if you are in severe pain it certainly makes sense to go to bed for a few days until the pain lessens. There is no evidence that specific exercise programs at this stage are better than simply carrying out normal activities.

If the pain is severe you will probably need to rest in bed. However, if the pain is so severe that you are unable to straighten up, you may have to lower yourself cautiously to the floor without altering the angle of your back. In any case you should avoid repeating any movement you think may have brought on the pain, or that causes it to intensify.

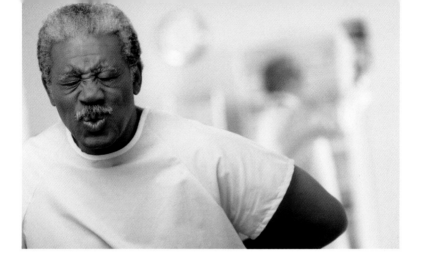

Acute pain is the kind that comes on suddenly and may be severe, causing you to stop whatever you are doing. You may well need to get yourself into a prone position, and should try to avoid movements that increase the pain.

Position There is no rule about which position you should adopt when you are in bed; lie in whatever position you find most comfortable, even though that may well not be lying flat. Often it is better if your hips and knees are flexed at about 90 degrees, which you can achieve with pillows or, if you are on the floor, with a chair under your legs. This is particularly likely to be helpful if the pain is mainly in the front of your thigh, as it is in some cases of disk prolapse affecting one of the higher lumbar levels. See lumbar disk prolapse (p.37).

The mattress Sitting up is usually painful and therefore should generally be avoided, although occasionally people find that it is more comfortable than lying down. Helpful friends may recommend a hard mattress or advise you to place boards underneath your existing mattress. This is seldom either necessary or desirable; unless your mattress sags badly it should be adequate as it is, and indeed, a very firm mattress may be more uncomfortable than a softer one. If your bed is really unsatisfactory you may be better off placing your mattress on the floor.

Turning over in bed is often difficult, especially if the bedclothes are heavy. It is better to keep the room warm rather than use too many blankets. To turn over in bed, draw your knees up and allow the weight of your legs to pull you over without twisting your spine.

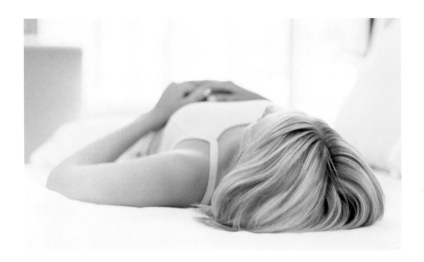

If pain is severe, you need to lie flat on a firm surface, which may be your bed, or even the floor.

Constipation

Getting to the lavatory may be a problem, but it is generally better to try to do so provided it is on the same floor and within reasonably easy reach. Alternative solutions such as bedpans, even if they are available, usually have more disadvantages than benefits for most people. It is likely that you will be constipated for the first few days, partly because of lack of movement, partly because of inhibition by pain, and sometimes because of medicines that your doctor may have prescribed. This is nothing to worry about and you need not do anything about it; it will sort itself out later, or you can try a stool softener.

Pain relief with medication

You will almost certainly need to have medicine to relieve the pain. Aspirin or acetaminophen may be enough if taken at the maximum permissible dosage; if not you will have to consult your doctor, who may prescribe one of the nonsteroidal anti-inflammatory drugs (NSAIDs), such as ibuprofen (Motrin). In spite of their name, their main action in this case is not to prevent inflammation but to relieve pain. If you have a history of stomach ulcers or bleeding these drugs, and aspirin, are unsuitable, so a different type may be prescribed. This may be one of the opium family, which the doctor may also prefer if the pain is very severe; these drugs tend to make constipation worse.

Pain relief without medication

Drugs are not the only way of relieving the pain. A hot water bottle may give relief. Perhaps rather surprisingly, cold applications may do so as well. A bag of frozen peas can work well, but remember that it is possible to suffer skin burns from cold as well as from heat. Prevent this by applying Vaseline or a damp towel between the skin and the ice pack, and do not leave it in place for more than about 15 or 20 minutes at a time. Both heat and cold seem to work by what is called counterirritation: that is, by stimulating the nerves going to the spinal cord in the affected region in such a way as to block the transmission of pain to the brain. This is an example of the gate theory at work. This is discussed in the next chapter (pp. 101–102).

Massage

It can help if someone massages your back, but this should be done gently, using some lubricating substance such as baby oil. There is no need to use any of the proprietary "pain relieving" creams, although you may do so if you wish. These mostly act as another form of counterirritant; they contain minor skin irritants that produce a feeling of local warmth by stimulating an increase in blood flow. A different type of cream contains NSAIDs, drugs similar to those taken by mouth, that act directly on the site of pain. But since the spine is placed too deeply for them to reach it, the effect is probably little different than if the same drug were taken by mouth. The risks of causing bleeding from the stomach are also similar.

Alternative treatments

You may wonder about seeking treatment from an alternative practitioner such as an osteopath, chiropractor, or acupuncturist. Even if you do not think of this yourself it is quite likely that a friend or relative will suggest it. Since it is probable that you will recover anyway given time, the main reason for trying one of these forms of treatment is to see if it will speed up the recovery process and get you backon your feet sooner than would otherwise be the case. Many people certainly report that they benefit from these forms of treatment, and although firm research evidence to support their use is difficult to produce, it may be reasonable to try. However, manipulation should not be used if there are signs of a disk prolapse, such as muscle weakness or loss of sensation, since it may make things worse. Acupuncture would be safe from this point of view but it will not, of course, cause a prolapsed disk to go back into place. Recovery can take place only in other ways, such as shrinkage of the disk material, which usually occurs naturally with time and patience.

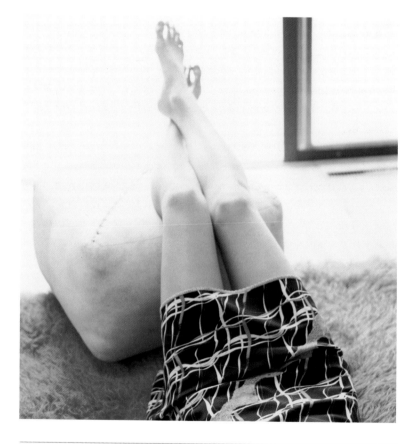

Raising your legs in this position may be more comfortable than lying completely flat. You should take up whichever position suits you best.

TENS: a safe alternative to drugs

Some people find relief from using a TENS (transcutaneous electrical nerve stimulation) machine. This is a method of applying a small electrical stimulation to the skin via conducting pads or electrodes. The machines are about the size of a cigarette pack and have one or more pairs of wires attached to them to conduct the current. They are battery-operated and quite safe to use (unless you have a cardiac pacemaker). They produce a mild tingling sensation in the skin. Pain relief usually begins soon after the machine is switched on and continues for as long as it is running. Relief tends to fade after the current is switched off, so patients may need to keep the machine running for long periods. It is quite possible to walk around and go to work while TENS is working. These machines are sold widely and are relatively cheap to buy. They do not work for everyone but, when they do, they provide a safe alternative to drugs. The nervous system adapts quickly to the stimulus and therefore the strength of the current has to be increased after a few minutes' use.

Initially patients should use the machine for at least an hour three times a day; alternatively, they can use it all day. Pain relief generally occurs soon after the machine is switched on; if it doesn't, the position of the electrodes or the setting of the controls should be altered. Trial and error are essential for success. Patients also need to understand that relief is often felt only while the stimulation is happening; if there is a carryover into the poststimulation time this is a bonus but it doesn't always occur.

The healing process

Acute back pain is likely to get better by itself, with or without treatment. If there are definite signs of nerve pressure causing sciatica, recovery may take longer but it is still likely to occur within a few weeks. Treatment is mainly intended to give pain relief while natural healing takes place. Manipulation or acupuncture may speed recovery, but high-velocity manipulation should be avoided if there are definite signs of sciatica with numbness and/or weakness. Remember that there are causes of sciatic-type pain that respond well to manipulation and are not caused by large disk protrusions that would be dangerous to compress with manipulation. But there are other techniques of manipulation that are non-force and effective, such as flexion distraction.

treating
chronic
back pain

Current research into how we feel pain suggests complex physical and psychological causes. Why is it that sometimes, even though the underlying problem appears to have been solved, pain remains? Often the symptoms of chronic back pain are, however, so severe and the causes so obvious that nothing short of minor or major surgery will do. In this chapter we look at some of the newer treatments that can provide long-term relief for patients. Some involve a simple injection, or simply facing your fears; others require more drastic action and, as in all forms of treatment, the results are not guaranteed.

Given the complexity of causation in chronic back pain, there is often no simple answer regarding treatment. The chance of finding a single abnormality that can be removed surgically, such as a prolapsed disk is slim, and the quest for a complete cure is often doomed. In many cases the sufferer needs to think more in terms of how to cope with the situation that exists.

Clearly a lot will depend on the frequency and severity of the pain. Some people experience bouts of pain that subside after a few days or weeks, allowing the sufferer to resume his or her normal activities. In such cases it is reasonable to take medicines to relieve the pain when it occurs, or perhaps use a TENS machine discussed in the previous chapter (p. 99), but otherwise to carry on as usual. When the pain is more or less continuous a different approach will probably be needed. The emphasis then should be as much on pain management as on cure. Treatments of this kind, called multidisciplinary rehabilitation, depend critically on new ideas about pain that have emerged in recent years.

New ideas about pain

Some patients continue to feel pain long after their original injury has healed. In the past many doctors thought that this meant patients were imagining their pain or even faking it. Now we know that pain is a great deal more complex than the simple model doctors used to rely on. This suggested that, if you injured yourself, the damaged area sent messages up the nerves and spinal cord to the brain, and a feeling of pain resulted. Once healing of the injury had occurred there should logically be no pain.

It is quite possible for genuine pain to persist for weeks, months, or even years after the original injury has healed. On the other hand, some severe injuries, for example, battle wounds, may cause no pain at all at the time they were inflicted.

Old pain versus new Pain is much more complex than the old model suggests. According to this idea, which was current for at least 300 years, pain depends on a signaling system rather like the bells in older houses, where one pulled on a rope which in turn pulled a wire that ran through the house to a board in the servants' quarters. Here it rang a bell and also activated a signal that showed in which room the rope had been pulled. In much the same way, an injury to some part of the body was supposed to send messages along the nerves to some part of the brain, which then recorded that the relevant part of the body had been damaged. But this rather simplistic model of pain perception is certainly inadequate.

The new view of pain stems from the work of two researchers in the 1970s, P.D. Wall and R. Melzack, who put forward what they called the gate theory. It works like this. Certain nerve cells in the spinal cord are capable of either decreasing or increasing the amount of pain information transmitted onward to the brain. Nerve impulses coming to the spinal cord via the large nerve fibers that carry the sense of touch tend to decrease this transmission; this explains the well-known experience of "rubbing it better" to relieve pain. Rubbing the skin, or stimulating it in other ways, tends to close the gates in the spinal cord and thus prevent the transmission of pain information to the brain. TENS machines (p.99) probably act in this way.

Not only nerves from the skin can have this effect. We now recognise that pathways also come down from centers in the brain to the gates in the spinal cord. Information carried in these pathways may either "open" the gates or "close" them. Many different factors can alter the amount and character of this information, including information from the parts of the brain concerned with consciousness.

Recent research has found that when pain persists different pathways are used, and the types of pain receptors and the biochemistry in the nervous system change. This means that chronic pain must be treated differently from acute pain. When pain first starts, a fairly simple pathway brings the painful sensation to our consciousness. But if the pain persists, another more complex pathway "opens up." This causes changes in blood flow and makes the nerves much more sensitive to a wide variety of stimuli. Elimination of the original problem may not be enough to stop the pain. Even if the problem is successfully treated these sensitized nerves can be easily re-ignited with reoccurrence of the whole pain syndrome. Therefore, treatment of these types of problems is more complex and often must include a variety of methods that attack the problem from several points of view.

Summary Feeling pain turns out to be a very complicated affair. It is influenced not only by the presence or the amount of damage to the body but a combination of many factors, some physical, some mental. And it is perfectly possible to have pain that is unrelated to tissue damage; pain can be, and often is, produced and even prolonged just by the activity of nerve cells in the spinal cord or brain. The gate theory, now widely accepted by pain specialists, sheds a great deal of light on how people's emotional state and attitude to their pain can alter the degree of pain they feel. Perception of pain is, to a considerable extent, a matter of attention to pain. The more you think about your pain, the worse it gets; conversely, by distracting yourself you can decrease the amount of pain you feel.

Multidisciplinary rehabilitation

The multidisciplinary approach draws on these insights and has several advantages. First, it widens the focus of treatment so that it looks, not just at pain, but at broader

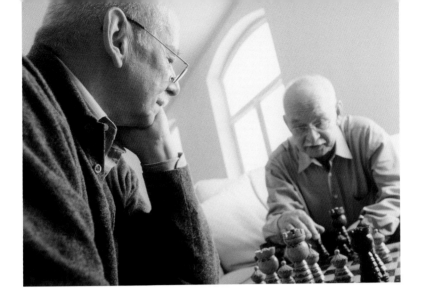

Distracting yourself by becoming absorbed in a good book or an engrossing game of chess may decrease the amount of pain you feel.

issues; this could be termed "treating the patient as a whole" in the true sense of that overused expression. Second, the shift from aiming to "cure" a patient toward trying to obtain the best adjustment possible is much more honest and realistic for chronic back pain sufferers. Third, the patient becomes very intimately involved in the process, since its success depends critically on his or her understanding and active participation. The patient changes from being the passive recipient of treatment to being an active partner. Although not everyone is willing or able to participate in schemes of this kind. Research has shown that they work well for those who are.

Cognitive-behavioral therapy This is an important part of the multidisciplinary approach. Cognitive-behavioral therapy (CBT) is not the same as the kind of psychotherapy that many people are more or less familiar with; it is not counseling. It is concerned mainly with the way that patients perceive their situation and the ideas and beliefs that they have about their backs.

For example, you may develop a fear of lifting after an occasion when you experienced pain when lifting, or someone – perhaps a doctor – may have told you that lifting can damage nerves in your spine. You may also become fearful if you have seen someone suffering acute back pain as the result of lifting.

Vicious circles This can set up a vicious circle of fear avoidance. You start to avoid all those situations that might involve lifting, and whenever you feel a slight twinge of pain you think that you must have made some unwise movement. This reinforces your fear, and thus you become locked into a vicious circle of fear and pain. Eventually you may not dare to bend over at all. And because maintenance of healthy disks and joints depends in part on exercising them, the avoidance of movement in itself makes your back worse (see "The Structure of the Back", the intervertebral disks, p. 18).

Fear of pain This may take various forms. Some patients do not recognize that they are afraid and simply say that they find certain movements or activities difficult to carry out. Others are not afraid of immediate pain but of pain that will occur later, perhaps the next day; or they may not be afraid of pain itself but rather of the injury, or reinjury, which they believe is connected to the pain.

The aim of CBT – and the other techniques used in the multidisciplinary approach to back pain – is to break this vicious circle of fear-pain avoidance. It is, in a sense, a form of education in which the patient participates. Just telling people that it is all right for them to perform a particular movement is not very effective. A better method is to teach them graded exercises. Much the best method, however, is to expose them gradually to whatever frightens them, such as a particular movement or activity.

Pain as a phobia For many patients, fear of back pain is a phobia like any other, and can be treated in much the same way. Treatment is by graded exposure to situations patients perceive as dangerous or threatening. This exposure is always introduced with a careful explanation of the fear-avoidance process, and uses the sufferer's symptoms, beliefs, and behaviors to illustrate how it works. This is quite similar to a graded exercise program, but with the critical difference that it is focused on the patient's particular concern.

EMG feedback Reeducation via graded exposure is often combined with other approaches to pain management. These might include physiotherapy, hypnosis, relaxation, and EMG feedback. The electrical activity in the patient's muscles is recorded and the information fed back to allow her or him to reduce the tension. Different centers combine these, and other methods, in different ways; there is no one fixed pattern. This can make it difficult to know which of the treatments is best, or whether it is the combination that works. A multifocal approach of this kind, however, can certainly be beneficial and represents a new and important approach to chronic back pain.

Nonsurgical interventions

Specialists have a range of possible treatments available to them. The minor, or non-surgical, interventions include injection therapy and traction.

Injection therapy An injection, usually a mixture of corticosteroid and local anesthetic, is given into the lower back in the lumbar or sacral region. The site of the injection may be the epidural space; that is, the space between the wall of the spinal canal and the epidural or outermost layer of the tissues covering the spinal cord and nerve roots; or it may be into the facet joints. It is usually done as an outpatient procedure and patients can go home after 20 or 30 minutes.

Other types of injection therapy are proliferative therapy and prolotherapy. Simple substances such as sugar, often combined with a local anesthetic are injected into damaged tissues. These substances act as local irritants. stimulating the tissue to proliferate, growing new tissue to repair the damaged tissue. The process will also destroy small nerve endings that cause pain but that serve little other purpose.

Traction therapy Traction is used to treat sciatica and neck pain. The spine is placed under tension by some form of weight apparatus, or simply by using gravity. The traction may be applied continuously or intermittently. Evidence that it works is somewhat mixed.

Surgery

Surgery is a major intervention and often a last resort, and includes rhizotomy and rhizolysis, intradiskal electrothermal therapy, nucleoplasty, discectomy, and lumbar fusion.

Rhizotomy and rhizolysis These are treatments in which nerve roots are cut or destroyed with the aim or reducing pain, although the actual cutting of a nerve root is very rare, except in cases of severe, intractable pain usually in terminally ill cancer patients. More common is a facet rhizotomy, done as an outpatient, in which the small nerve at the back of the facet joint between the vertebrae is destroyed; this relieves pain temporarily and may be repeated.

IDET (intradiskal electrothermal therapy) This is performed by placing a needle into the disk and then passing a heating catheter through it. The catheter is used to heat the annulus of the disk, causing destruction of painful nerve endings and shrinking of the disk itself. This is done as an outpatient procedure. The disk heals after two months.

Surgery is usually a last resort in the treatment of chronic back pain, but it can be valuable in certain cases.

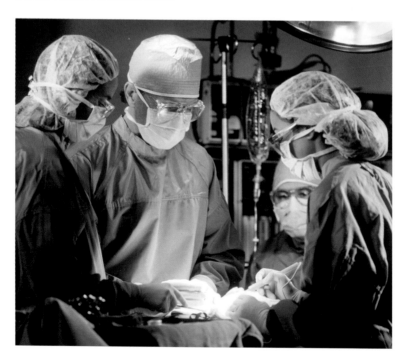

Nucleoplasty This is when a needle is placed into the disk and an electrode is passed through it. As it is passed through the disk it is heated destroying disk material and thereby shrinking the disk.

Discectomy This is a surgical treatment to remove disk material (*nucleus pulposus*) that has escaped and is pressing on nerve roots. The surgeon opens the spine and removes the disk material. Some techniques require more opening up of the back than others: in laminectomy part or all of the neural arch (made up of two *laminas*, hence the term) is cut away; fenestration is a more limited technique in which no bone is cut away. Some surgeons have developed microsurgical procedures in which only a small opening is made and the operation takes well under an hour. Laser discectomy has also been tried but there is little information available about its effectiveness.

Surgical discectomy for carefully selected patients with sciatica, due to lumbar disk prolapse, gives faster pain relief than waiting for natural recovery. Whether the long-term results are better or worse is still unclear. Surgeries that cut away bone can cause instability that may later be the cause of severe pain and eventually result in the need for a spinal fusion.

Indications for discectomy are: severe pain that persists after epidural injection and/or rest; bladder symptoms that indicate a catastrophically huge disk protrusion; and progressive neurologic loss, especially foot drop for a L-5 (5th lumbar vertebra) root compression, although some physicians would argue that surgery does not help this latter situation.

Lumbar fusion This is performed when there is not enough room for the nerve roots owing to arthritis of the facet joints, instability of the spine, spondylolisthesis, or when the disks themselves are the source of pain. Often these patients have back pain without leg pain. This kind or surgery is quite complicated and is therefore reserved for specific difficult situations.

All these surgical treatments can help pain. As with any operation, back surgery does unfortunately have a failure rate. When an operation is unsuccessful this poses a difficult problem for both patient and surgeon. Any of these surgeries can result in scarring of the dura or the nerve roots. This is a severe and often intractable cause of pain. Second and even third operations are sometimes undertaken but the results are considerably worse and the technical difficulties are greater.

It's rather different for neck pain because the spinal cord makes surgery more difficult. The evidence shows that surgery for neck problems helps in pain, weakness, and sensory loss in the short term, but after a year it suggests that there is no real difference between patients who have had surgery and those who simply wore an immobilizing collar.

Nerve root irritation in the neck, causing pain, often settles by itself in four to six months, so surgery is not indicated for this and pain-relieving treatments like those used for the lumbar spine can be used while waiting for spontaneous recovery.

It's rather different for neck pain because the spinal cord makes surgery more difficult. The evidence shows that surgery for neck problems helps in pain, weakness, and sensory loss in the short term, but after a year it suggest that there is no real difference between patients who have had surgery and those who simply wore an immobilizing collar. It is therefore unclear whether the risks of operation for neck symptoms outweigh any possible benefits.

Summary

Various treatments may be used for back pain, both in the acute phase and more chronic situations. In any individual case one has to balance the possible risks

TREATING OSTEOPOROSIS

Hormone replacement therapy (HRT) increases bone density if given at menopause, but the risks and benefits of using it need to be assessed in each individual case. HRT needs to be continued for 5–10 years to be effective. Raloxifene is similar to HRT but only affects osteoporosis; it does not affect hot flushes. If HRT is unsuitable for any reason, alternative treatments exist. Calcitonin is one, and there is a newer range of drugs called the bisphosphonates (alendronate, etidronate, risedronate) which decrease the risk of fractures.

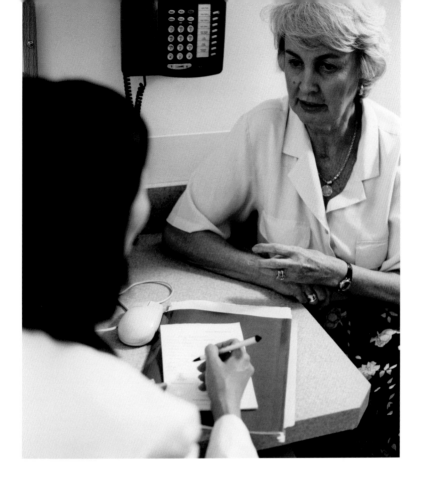

Your doctor is usually the first port of call when suffering from back pain, and can advise you about the need to seek further advice or treatment from a specialist.

and benefits carefully. Patients should discuss the pros and cons with their specialists and their doctors in some detail before deciding.

The treatments for mainly chronic back pain are all more or less focused on finding identifiable things that have gone wrong in your back. When treatments work they are fine, but unfortunately many patients have chronic back pain that cannot be helped in these ways.

At this stage many of them may consider one of the alternative therapies that is the subject of the next three chapters.

TREATING CHRONIC BACK PAIN   **109**

therapies
and
therapists

As we saw in the discussion of acute back pain, you may choose to seek alternative treatment as soon as an attack is experienced; this is more likely to be the case if there have been previous episodes of pain in which an alternative approach has helped. More frequently, however, sufferers take this route when conventional treatment has failed. There is in any case an increase in the popularity of alternative treatment, which means that, if you have significant back pain, it is likely that you will think of trying it simply because it is so often mentioned in the media and appears to work for many people. Indeed, a friend or relative will probably suggest it.

A great many forms of alternative treatments are available, and the range of options can be bewildering. However, there is a fairly small group that is generally regarded as "central" and for that reason has received more attention from researchers. For the same reason there is in many countries a move toward regulation of these therapies; in fact, osteopathy and chiropractic are already regulated in Britain, and other therapies are set to follow in the near future.

This central group of therapies is sometimes referred to as "the big four": manipulation (osteopathy and chiropractic), acupuncture, herbal medicine, and homeopathy. Manipulation and acupuncture differ from the others in being physical treatments; they are therefore the most likely to be used by back pain sufferers.

Although the "big four" are still classed as alternative therapies there is a definite trend for them to move into the conventional sphere, and the boundary between alternative and mainstream is becoming increasingly blurred. For example, many physiotherapists use manipulative techniques borrowed from osteopathy, and an increasing number also use acupuncture. Doctors are becoming increasingly interested in acupuncture, though mainly in its modern (medical) form rather than the traditional Chinese version. It is possible that some of the injection techniques (see p.105) used to treat back pain work in much the same way as acupuncture. This tendency to increasing use of alternative techniques by mainstream practitioners seems likely to continue, and indeed to accelerate.

Many conventional physiotherapists and doctors use manipulation and acupuncture techniques in their practices today.

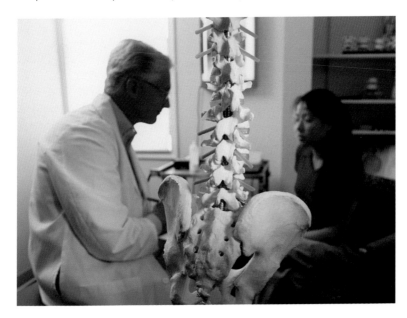

Choosing an alternative practitioner

In most cases the first step should be to ask the advice of your GP. These days an increasing number of general practitioners have trained in homeopathy, acupuncture, or osteopathy. If not, your GP may be able to recommend someone whom they trust, and some GPs have complementary therapists working part-time in their practices. It is no longer considered unethical for doctors to refer their patients for alternative treatment provided they retain overall responsibility for their care.

Patients are sometimes afraid that their doctor will resent being asked about such matters and it is true that some are strongly prejudiced against all forms of alternative treatment, but such doctors are becoming rarer these days. It is however possible that your doctor will advise against such treatment in your case, and there may be a good medical reason for this. For example, if your spine were unstable for some reason it would be unwise to have manipulation, and if you were taking anticoagulant drugs, acupuncture would need to be performed with care, if at all.

In some cases it may not be strictly necessary to ask your doctor's opinion. If you have a long history of back pain that has been fully investigated in the past, no harm will be done if you try a different approach on your own. Even in such a case, however, it would be better to inform your doctor of your decision, and the practitioner you consult may want to let your doctor know what he plans to do. This has to be with your permission, however, and you are entitled to refuse.

If you do decide to find a practitioner yourself, the best way to do so is by personal recommendation from someone whose opinion you trust. Only if all fails should you resort to picking a name at random from the telephone directory or similar lists. If you do have to do this, at least make sure that the therapist you choose has evidence of adequate training and professional standards. This is sometimes difficult in the case of those professions that are not at present statutorily regulated.

Telling your doctor

It may not be essential to get your doctor's approval. For example, if you have a long history of back pain for which you have already been investigated, no harm will be done if you decide to seek alternative treatment on your own initiative. Even in such a case, however, it would be better to tell your doctor, and the practitioner you consult probably should let him or her know, though this must be with your permission and you are entitled to refuse.

In the United Kingdom, some treatments such as homeopathy and acupuncture are available to some extent on the NHS, though this is not the case in all areas. Many physiotherapists use manipulative techniques or acupuncture as part of their standard treatment. However, you may well find that you have to pay. There is a bewildering choice, and not all forms of treatment are regulated at present.

Regulation

Osteopathy, chiropractic, and acupuncture are now licensed in the United States and herbal treatment is set to follow in the next few years. Chiropractic education in the United States is monitored by the Council on Chiropractic Education, which in turn is overseen by the Department of Education. Four years of training in basic and clinical science with National and State Board exams have to be undertaken in order to practice chiropractic in the United States. Osteopathic physicians are fully licensed physicians who can perform surgery and do anything else that M.D.s can do. They will also have had special training in manipulative medicine.

If a treatment is regulated, practitioners will, you can be sure, have professional qualifications and insurance. Otherwise, the old rule of caveat emptor (let the buyer beware) applies. See "Useful Organizations" p. 140.

Time and cost

Before agreeing to treatment you should inquire about cost and the expected number of treatments, so you know what you are letting yourself in for. It is impossible for a therapist to tell you exactly how many treatments will be required; this naturally varies from case to case, but you should not be asked to sign up in advance for a specified number of treatments. As a general rule, you should expect to see at least some benefit after two or three physical treatments such as osteopathy, chiropractic, or acupuncture. Homeopaths sometimes warn that improvement takes time, but in that case the consultations should be at fairly long intervals. Ask about the likelihood of success. Again, this is often difficult to predict, but be wary of overconfident statements. No form of therapy can guarantee success, and it would be wrong for any practitioner to promise a complete cure.

physical
therapies

Most people with back pain first think of trying some form of physical treatment and this is sensible, since in many cases the pain will be due to a mechanical problem of some kind in the back. Some therapies, such as osteopathy and chiropractic, are generally thought of as treatments designed to put right things that have gone wrong, perhaps by moving the spinal joints into better alignment. Others, such as the Alexander Technique, are more concerned with re-education of the way in which we use our bodies and are probably mainly applicable to long-term prevention of problems. However, this distinction is by no means absolute and almost all practitioners will include an element of prevention in their approach to spinal problems.

Osteopathy and chiropractic

It is convenient to consider osteopathy and chiropractic together, even though their origins are somewhat different, because the techniques they use have a lot in common. Osteopathy derives from the work of an American doctor, Andrew Taylor Still (1828–1912); chiropractic from that of a Canadian, David Henry Palmer (1845–1913), who was not a doctor. As a result of this historical difference, doctors today sometimes train as osteopaths but hardly ever as chiropractors. The theories underlying the two treatments in their early years were different and, even today, chiropractors tend to use X-rays more than osteopaths.

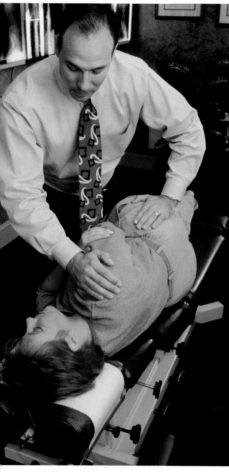

An osteopath manipulating the spine. Although firm pressure is used at times, the treatment is not generally painful.

Patients often expect that treatment by either type of practitioner will consist mainly of moving their spine or limbs, often with an audible "crack," but manipulation of this kind is only part of the treatment and may not even be the main part. The aim is not just to correct misalignments of joints or vertebrae, but to assess how well the patient's body is functioning in relation to everyday living. Patients are generally expected to help themselves by modifying their lifestyle and activities. Contrary to what you may have heard, manipulation is generally not painful or violent; mostly it is gentle and pain-free.

Manipulation is generally safe, although there are certain recognized dangers. For example, it would be unsafe to manipulate a spine that contained cancerous areas or that was affected by rheumatoid arthritis in the neck. Registered osteopaths and chiropractors are trained to look out for these problems.

The assessment The exact course of consultation with an osteopath or chiropractor is likely to vary somewhat from one practitioner to another, but they generally begin by making a detailed assessment of the way you stand and move. Differences in the height of the hipbones and in the location of skin folds and other features can indicate abnormalities of various kinds. These may be due to recently acquired back problems or may themselves be the cause. Osteopaths frequently diagnose a short leg, either left or right; the consequent tilt in the pelvis is thought to be a cause of strain in the spine and hence of back pain. Sometimes the insertion of a simple lift in a shoe will give relief, although the reason for this is not always obvious. Minor degrees of leg shortening are not easy to detect without the help of standing-up X-rays, which are not routinely taken. The adaptability of the spine should not be underestimated, therefore leg shortening does not necessarily give rise to any symptoms.

While most chiropractors and osteopaths in the United States perform detailed physicals (checking pulse and blood pressure, a neurological exam, postural exam, myofascial exam, and orthopedic testing), not all osteopaths or chiropractors make this detailed assessment; some prefer to treat the main problem quite quickly and in such cases the consultation may be brief. More often, however, the preliminary discussion of your symptoms will last 5 or 10 minutes; then there will be a physical examination lasting about the same time, and then 10 to 15 minutes' treatment, followed by explanation and advice. Depending on your progress, further treatments might require examinations on each occasion, or, if you are recovering well, there might be more time for discussion and advice about preventing recurrence.

How many treatments? Although it is unrealistic to expect a dramatic and complete cure from just one treatment, there should normally be at least some improvement after two or three sessions. If no improvement has occurred by then it may not be worth continuing with that particular practitioner.

Most patients should expect to receive somewhere between two to four weeks of treatment. After this, most people are either cured or have reached a plateau beyond which continued treatment may produce little further improvement quickly. At this point treatment should stop unless or until a relapse occurs, although some practitioners advise an occasional maintenance treatment to keep problems at bay. This treatment pattern is common to most forms of physical therapy and acupuncture.

Massage techniques

Massage is probably as old as humanity, and is likely an extension of the instinctive reaction to rub a place that hurts. In some countries, such as India and Iran, it is customary to ask a relative to walk on your back in bare feet to relieve muscular aches and pains. Many people find this pleasurable in itself, whether or not they are in pain.

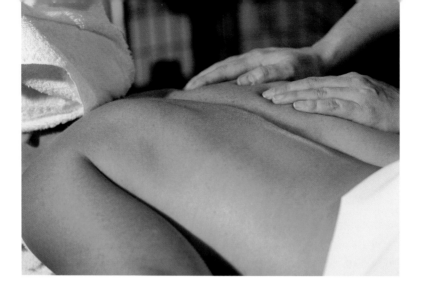

Massage is probably the oldest form of manual therapy and is still the most widely used alternative treatment today.

Many systematic massage techniques exist. In Scandinavia it is part of the standard training of physiotherapists. One form, aromatherapy, uses scented "essential oils" that are rubbed into the skin and are said to have therapeutic effects; this is really a combination of herbalism and massage.

The vigor with which massage is performed varies according to the therapist. Some use very gentle, pain-free touch methods, while others go for firmer pressure that may be moderately painful. At the extreme is the technique known as Rolfing.

Rolfing This type of manipulation or massage is named after Ida Rolf (1896–1979). She was a doctor of biochemistry who began to develop this method in the 1940s, although it was not until the 1960s, when she moved to Esalen in California, that she began to train students. The Rolf Institute was established in the 1970s and now has branches in several countries.

Rolfing aims to correct imbalances in the muscles and in the connective tissue, which is found throughout the body and which acts as support and "packing," covering muscles, nerves, and other structures. In the course of her work Rolf came to believe that emotional states become locked into our bodies and can create postural changes. Thus we speak of someone being "bowed with grief" or "hunched against the blows of fate."

Rebalancing the physical body using Rolfing techniques involves firm kneading of the tissues all over the body. This can be painful and may also release locked-in emotions, so that patients may laugh or cry for long periods. Phenomena of this kind are not unique to Rolfing and they also occur with other forms of manipulation such as those employed by physiotherapists, osteopaths, and chiropractors, and also during acupuncture.

Hellerwork This technique was founded by Joseph Heller who originally studied at the Rolf Institute, but later developed his own methods based on deep-tissue massage and postural reeducation. It includes talking with the subject to increase their awareness about their emotional attitudes. The Hellerwork handbook can be downloaded from the internet (see "Useful Organizations" p.140).

Acupuncture needles may be placed along the spine to relieve pain. The picture shows the traditional approach, using many needles; some practitioners use fewer needles, sometimes only one.

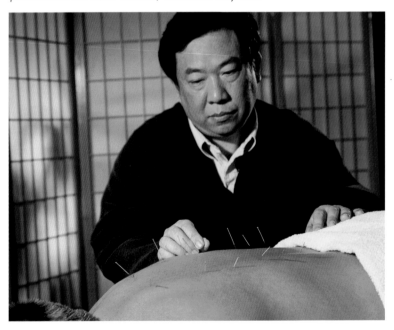

Acupuncture

Acupuncture is a Western term meaning the treatment of conditions through the insertion of solid needles. In this respect it differs from injection therapy, which uses hollow needles. Other terms used occasionally, such as "dry needling" or "intramuscular stimulation," refer to the same thing.

Acupuncture originated in China, where it has a long history going back at least 2,000 years, although many of the ideas in current practice have a later origin. No one knows how acupuncture began, although it may have developed from tattooing. Interestingly, the "ice man," whose 4,000-year-old body was recently discovered in the Alps, has tattoo marks in his back. Could this indicate acupuncture for back pain?

Acupuncture has long been practiced in different forms in other Far Eastern countries such as Japan, Korea, and Vietnam, and it came to the West as early as the end of the 17th century. It was quite widely practiced in a number of European countries, including France and England, in the early 19th century, however, the modern surge of interest dates from President Nixon's visit to China in 1972, when doctors saw operations being carried out using acupuncture instead of conventional anesthesia. Since then there has been a considerable increase in interest in acupuncture on the part of doctors and other health professionals in the West, as part of the growing popularity of alternative medicine.

In the West mainstream doctors have always tended to use acupuncture independently of the ancient Chinese theories, and this is still the case. At present, therefore, there are two main versions of acupuncture current in the West: traditional Chinese and modern or medical. The differences are more theoretical than practical, since both, after all, use needles, but there are some practical differences as well.

Traditional acupuncture This is based on the idea that there is a subtle "substance" or "energy" called chi (also written qi), which flows through the body in special channels or pathways (the "meridians"). Scattered along these channels are the sites at which acupuncture is performed (the "points"). The concept of chi is linked to that of yin-yang polarity; the theory posits two mutually opposed, yet complementary, tendencies in the universe and also in our bodies. Health is held to depend on a correct balance between yin and yang, and hence on maintaining the flow of chi in a balanced way. Too much or too little chi in an organ gives rise to disease. Acupuncture is said to work by regulating the flow of chi. The acupuncturist is thus a kind of engineer, controlling the flow of chi along its pathways like raising or lowering lock gates in a canal system. Contrary to how some people think of acupuncture, there is nothing mystical about this.

Modern acupuncture Modern acupuncture recognizes that many of the phenomena described by the traditional acupuncturists are real but seeks to explain them in different terms. So, in modern terms acupuncture acts via the conventionally understood nervous system; there is no need to accept the existence of the "meridians," chi, and so forth. The nervous system influences other systems, such as the endocrine (ductless glands) and immune systems, so it may be possible to explain the many effects of acupuncture in a modern context.

Modern acupuncture does not accept the traditional theories that disease is due to yin-yang imbalance; the ordinary disease categories used in modern medicine are recognized. Most modern practitioners make use of trigger point ideas (see p. 44) to a greater or lesser extent. Many doctors, physiotherapists, osteopaths, chiropractors, podiatrists, and nurses who use acupuncture do so in a modern way, although some do practice the traditional version to a greater or lesser degree.

Traditional versus modern acupuncture The treatment you experience may differ according to the kind of practitioner you consult. A traditionalist and modernist will be interested in different aspects of your history and make use of certain special examinations, notably the appearance of the tongue and the character of the pulse. Traditional treatment will usually involve inserting a considerable number of needles, which are left in for about 20 minutes. The acupuncturist may stimulate the needles at times, either manually or by means of electricity. There may be some pain but it should not be excessive.

Modern acupuncturists, however, use much shorter needle insertion times, perhaps only a couple of minutes or less. This may seem surprising to anyone who has experienced the traditional method but there is no evidence that it is any more or less effective. Often, also, fewer needles are inserted; perhaps no more than four and sometimes just one. Again, the effect may be just as great.

Risks Unlike most other forms of alternative treatment, acupuncture involves piercing of the skin. This carries a risk of infection, which might be by bacteria causing inflammation, abscesses, or blood poisoning, or might be by a virus such as hepatitis or even AIDS; although there have been no confirmed cases of AIDS caused by acupuncture, it is possible, since cases of Hepatitis B infection through unsterilized needles have been reported in the United Kingdom. Today, however, all responsible acupuncture practitioners use disposable needles, which makes the transmission of any form of infection virtually impossible.

Another risk is of damage to underlying organs and other structures. In practice, the biggest danger is of puncturing the lungs, causing a collapse called a pneumothorax. Provided the acupuncturist is trained in anatomy this risk is very small.

At present, acupuncture is unregulated in many countries, including Britain, although this is set to change. It is regulated in the United States. You should also make sure that anyone from whom you receive acupuncture is either registered with one of the existing professional acupuncture bodies (see "Useful Organizations" p.140) or is a registered health professional.

To put all this in perspective: although there are recognized risks in acupuncture, provided it is performed by a suitably trained therapist with an adequate knowledge of anatomy the dangers are probably smaller than those of taking some of the medications, such as NSAIDs, that are often used to treat back pain. According to recent surveys in Britain, the incidence of unwanted effects following acupuncture is very low.

Acupuncture should generally be avoided in pregnancy because there is a theoretical risk that it will induce a miscarriage, particularly in the first three months. The lower back is one of the "forbidden areas" in pregnancy so it is inappropriate to treat backaches in pregnancy.

Success rates As with most forms of alternative medicine, it is difficult to obtain accurate estimates of the probability of success, because there have been too few good-quality studies. Much will depend on the nature of the individual's problem. As we discussed in the causes of chronic back pain (see "Symptoms and their Causes pp. 24–47), a patient's mood, life circumstances, and employment may all be influential, and where these are significant factors acupuncture is less likely to be successful. Contrary to what might be expected, acupuncture generally works best when there is some identifiable physical cause for the pain. For example, it can help in back pain due to ankylosing spondylitis (see p. 42), osteoarthritis (see p. 29), or osteoporosis (see p. 39). However, it is important to understand that acupuncture in this context is a treatment for pain rather than for the underlying disease; it is therefore unlikely to help where there is an anatomical problem such as a prolapsed lumbar disk pressing on a nerve root (see p. 37).

Ear acupuncture There are some specialized forms of acupuncture, of which the best known is ear acupuncture (auriculotherapy). It claims there is a map of the body in the ear, with the head represented at the bottom of the ear and the spine running up the outside; the legs and feet are at the top. This resembles the way these areas are represented in the motor and sensory areas in the brain.

Practitioners of ear acupuncture treat pain by needling the area of the ear corresponding to the part of the body that is affected. There is little reliable research about the effectiveness of ear acupuncture compared with body acupuncture. Therapists who claim to treat nicotine addiction and obesity with acupuncture generally use the ear, and ear acupuncture has formed part of some drug control programs. Little good evidence exists that this form of treatment has more than a placebo effect.

One problem with ear acupuncture, which is acknowledged even by people who favor it, is that its effects often last for only a short time. To get around this difficulty some therapists leave small needles in place for a week or more, but this poses the risk of infection entering the body via the needle site. There have been rare cases of infection of the heart valves (bacterial endocarditis) due to this practice. One alternative method, which is safe, is to fix tiny balls in place which exert pressure on the relevant sites in the ear.

Acupressure and Shiatsu These treatments are based on much the same theories as traditional Chinese acupuncture and use the same concepts of "meridians" and "points" but the treatment is given with finger pressure rather than needles. Both treatments use similar techniques; Shiatsu is the Japanese version. It is possible to apply pressure in a "modern" way, using concepts based on trigger

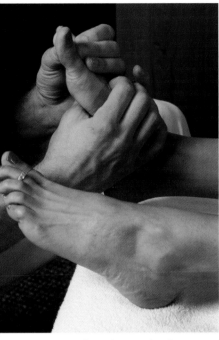

Reflexology involves applying pressure to the soles of the feet, which are thought to contain a map of the body.

points (see p. 44) rather than on traditional, Oriental theories (see pp. 119–120).

The obvious advantages of finger pressure compared with needles are that there is no risk of infection and those who fear needles need not worry. Indeed, patients can apply finger pressure to themselves. However, pressure techniques of this kind are not necessarily less painful than needling and indeed may be more painful. Generally, the relief is shorter lasting, although pressure can of course be applied as frequently as necessary.

Reflexology This has something in common with both Shiatsu and ear acupuncture, in that it makes use of finger pressure that is applied to the soles of the feet, which are also believed to contain a map of the body. There are claims that reflexology was used in ancient times in the East, but modern origins date from the work of Dr. W. Fitzgerald in the 1920s. There is little scientific evidence for its efficacy, although many patients do find that it helps.

Postural therapies

These include the Alexander Technique, Feldenkrais, and yoga, for which back problem sufferers claim varying results.

Alexander Technique This derives from the work of F. Matthias Alexander (1869–1955), an Australian actor at the end of the 19th century. The Alexander Technique began as a method of voice training for singers and actors, but the students found that it was helping other problems as well and eventually it evolved to become a more general procedure for improving the way the body functions as

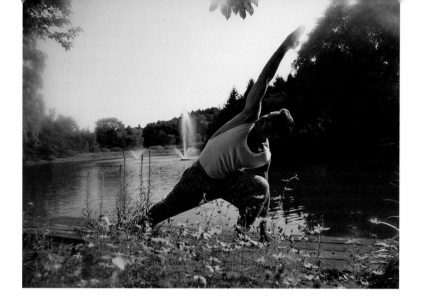

Yoga is an ancient Indian system in which postures are held for a certain time. Some back sufferers find it helpful, but a good teacher is essential.

a whole. Symptoms such as low-back pain are seen as one aspect of a wider failure of proper coordination.

The Alexander Principle implies that most of us have built up faulty patterns of movement that have become second nature, so that they feel "right" even though they are not. An Alexander student is taught a way of stopping and changing these habits by being guided through a set of basic movements. By repeating these, the student is supposed to reeducate his or her internal mechanisms of coordination. The technique does not involve exercises and differs in principle from manipulation and similar methods. It is claimed to be particularly suitable for people with chronic pain as well as those suffering from stress.

Although there have been attempts in recent years to adapt the teaching to group work, the technique is usually taught on an individual basis. Lessons last between half an hour and an hour, but there is no fixed number of sessions. Trainee teachers receive 1,600 or more hours of training over three or more years.

Feldenkrais The Feldenkrais method is described as a "unique and sophisticated approach to human understanding, learning, and change." It was developed by Moshe Feldenkrais (1904–1984), who was a scientist, physicist, and engineer as well as a judo instructor. It is claimed to improve posture, flexibility, coordination, self-image, and to alleviate muscular tension and pain. It has two components: "Awareness Through Movement" consists of verbally directed, gentle exercise lessons involving sophisticated movement sequences; "Functional Integration" uses specific skilled manipulation and passive movement.

Yoga This ancient Indian regime has been popular on and off for many years in the West and is undergoing a surge of enthusiasm thanks to its espousal by a number of high-profile celebrities. In its original form yoga had eight parts and was linked to traditions of seeking spiritual enlightenment, but most Westerners encounter it in its physical form as a series of postures called asanas. These are not exercises in the ordinary sense; indeed, one consists simply in lying flat on one's back! Each posture is held for a certain time.

Various benefits are claimed for yoga and it is claimed to be beneficial for back pain sufferers. However, such claims have to be interpreted with caution, because some of the postures presuppose a degree of spinal flexibility which Westerners, especially those of a certain age, don't usually have. Some, such as the shoulder stand, are definitely to be avoided by people with stiff spines. Not everyone enjoys yoga, but people who do may find that it helps their backs. However, it is essential to learn from an experienced teacher who knows how to adapt the method to meet the needs of people with vulnerable spines. At no time should students ever force themselves to achieve positions that they find difficult.

Pilates Exercise is often supervised by a physiotherapist, perhaps as part of a multidisciplinary approach (see pp. 102–105). A fashionable approach for back patients (and others) is Pilates, named after Joseph Pilates, a German in the 1920s who devised a series of movements that are carried out against resistance on a machine that uses spring loading. It was originally used by ballet dancers but now, thanks to a lot of publicity from certain high-profile celebrities, it is being taken up by a wide range of people. Like other specialized forms of movement and exercise, Pilates needs to be supervised by a competent instructor if it is to be safe, and you should attend classes to become proficient in the technique.

natural
therapies

The treatments described in this chapter are of two main
types. Some, such as homeopathy and herbal medicine,
make use of medicines that are mainly taken by mouth.
This may seem similar to conventional pharmacology,
but the difference is that these alternative medicines are
prescribed as much on the patient's general and often
psychological characteristics as on symptoms such as pain.
The second type of treatments contains psychological
methods of various kinds, most of which depend in one
way or another on relaxation. Most, however, would claim
to be more profound than mere relaxation and seek to
produce profound psychophysical changes.

Herbal medicine

Advocates of herbal medicines claim that when the whole plant is used the various
components interact with one another to give better results than when the "active
principle" is isolated and used alone, as in modern pharmacology.

Until surprisingly recently, the only medicines available to doctors were herbal.
Herbs have been used for their medicinal properties for thousands of years, and
each culture has developed unique and sophisticated ways of using plants to treat
human ailments. Scientists started extracting and isolating chemicals from plants in the
18th century, and mainstream medicine still uses plants as the basis for 25 percent
of all medicines prescribed.

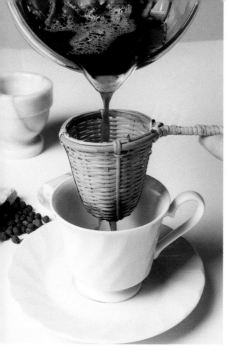

Until the 20th century most medicines were herbal and even today many medicines are derived from herbs. There are several different herbal traditions in use today. The medicines often come in the form of a tincture or extract, while some can be brewed as a tea.

With the advent of the modern pharmaceutical industry most herbal medicines ceased to be used, at least in their original form, and they were left in the hands of nonmedical prescribers who need not have had any formal training. Herbal medicine is still unregulated in Britain, and is largely unregulated in the United States, but this is set to change as new legislation is planned in the next few years.

One striking development in recent years has been the setting up of clinics of Chinese and Indian medicine. China and India have a long history of using herbs, some of which have been validated by modern research. The growth in availability of Eastern medicines in the West has, however, been problematic: sometimes the identification of imported plants has been incorrect and sometimes the medicines have been adulterated with other substances including modern pharmaceuticals as well as lead and mercury.

The National Institute of Medicinal Herbalists accredits practitioners who complete three- or four-year university degrees in herbal medicine. These practitioners have a thorough grounding in all the basic sciences of medicine (including anatomy, physiology, and pathology), but they specialize in using herbal therapeutics.

Risks Because herbal medicines are at present unregulated, patients are free to treat themselves with products bought over the counter or on the Internet, and many do so. This may be a tempting route if you suffer from chronic back pain that has failed to respond to conventional treatment but caution is needed.

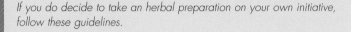

If you do decide to take an herbal preparation on your own initiative, follow these guidelines.

■ *Find out as much as you can about the effects of what you are taking and do not exceed the recommended dose.*

■ *Tell your doctor what you are taking, especially if you are also taking conventional medication. This may interact with the herbal medicine. This is particularly important if you are to have an anesthetic; some anesthetics become much more powerful if a patient is also taking certain herbal preparations. This could be dangerous.*

■ *Avoid taking more than one kind of herbal substance at a time, and keep careful note of any effects it may produce.*

■ *Read the labels carefully and check if the preparation has received any kind of official approval. In the United States the designation USP (United States Pharmacopeia) means that the medicine has an approved use and was manufactured according to certain standards. The designation NF (National Formulary) means that the medicine does not have a USP-approved use but was manufactured according to the same standards of quality and purity.*

■ *If you are pregnant or breast-feeding, don't take any herbal medicines without first consulting your doctor.*

■ *Don't expect immediate results. Read the label to see how long you need to take it before it has an effect. Be cautious about taking any medicine for long periods without professional advice.*

■ *Medicines manufactured in Europe and the United States are generally produced to a high standard and are regulated regarding quality and strength. This is not necessarily true of those coming from India or China, and it is prudent to be cautious in using them.*

First, there is little reliable information about either the safety or effectiveness of many of the products on sale. There is a widespread but mistaken belief that, because something is "natural," it is also safe. Remember that there are many highly poisonous substances in the natural world.

And remember that just because a substance has been used as a medicine for many hundreds of years, this does not necessarily mean that it is safe. If, for example, an herbal medicine caused cancer to develop only many years after it had been taken, this might well not have been picked up by practitioners in the past.

Second, there is still little standardization of the medicines on sale, either regarding quality or potency. Two preparations produced by different manufacturers may contain markedly different quantities of the active substances, and indeed, the nature and properties of these substances may not always be known.

Other natural products

Many patients find benefit from taking glucosamine or chrondroitin for osteoarthritis. Glucosamine is an amino sugar and chrondroitin is a carbohydrate component of cartilage; both are produced naturally by the body. When used as medicines, glucosamine is derived from shellfish shells and chondroitin is generally made from cow cartilage. Human studies show that both compounds are able to relieve the pain of arthritis and improve functioning with none of the unwanted effects of conventional drugs such as NSAIDs; they also seem to slow the progression of joint damage in osteoarthritis. A major research study on glucosamine is currently in progress and should provide useful information when it is finished. In the meantime it could certainly be reasonable to give these products a trial for a few months, but shop carefully regarding prices because these vary widely.

Homeopathy

Homeopathy is a system of medicine that developed in the late 18th and early 19th centuries thanks to the work of a German doctor, Samuel Christian Hahnemann (1755–1843). He became disillusioned with the medicine of his day, which was both ineffective and dangerous. A chance observation led him to formulate his own form of treatment, which he called homeopathy and which was based on the idea of similarity between the effects of the medicine and the symptoms of the patient.

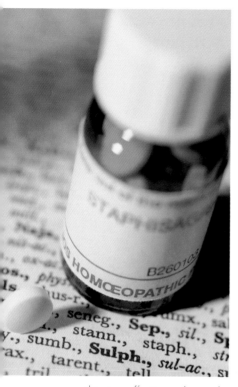

Homeopathic medicines are usually highly diluted and therefore mostly free from toxic affects. Accurate diagnosis is however necessary to make sure that homeopathy is appropriate in a particular case.

For example, a child with a fever would probably have a flushed, dry skin and might be delirious. These symptoms are similar to those produced by *belladonna* (deadly nightshade), so belladonna might be the treatment for a child with scarlet fever. For back pain the remedy might be *rhus toxicodendron* (poison ivy), because this produces muscle and joint pains in volunteers who take it by mouth.

Another of Hahnemann's innovations, and probably the one that has most strongly captured the public imagination, was his use of very small doses. These, he claimed, were almost as effective as larger doses; and later he came to believe that they were a great deal more effective. He believed that not only was the dilution important, but also vigorous shaking (succussion). Modern homeopathic medicines are still used in dilutions prepared with succussion, though now they are mostly prepared by machine rather than by hand, and the degree of dilution is often much greater than in Hahnemann's day.

The dilutions are made by taking one part of the crude substance, typically in a tincture, and mixing it with 9 or 99 parts water. When the dilution is one part in 10, the letter X is placed after the number – for example, 6X indicates six stages of serial dilution. When the dilution is one part in 100, the letter C is placed after the number of dilutions. This process reduces the amount of crude material present, but simultaneously seems to increase the remedy's healing power.

Homeopathy spread very widely during Hahnemann's lifetime and in the years following his death. It became particularly popular in the United States shortly after the end of the Civil War, but had virtually disappeared by the early 20th century. It is now beginning to revive. Today homeopathy is practiced throughout the world, both by doctors trained in homeopathy and by practitioners without a conventional medical qualification. As with herbal medicine, patients are free to buy the medicines for themselves, and many do so.

Low risk Because homeopathy nearly always uses very small doses there is almost no danger of drug-related side effects such as may occur with conventional or herbal medication. Theoretically, homeopathic medicines are capable of causing "aggravations" (worsening) of the symptoms from which patients suffer, but in practice these are very rare and may be almost entirely attributable to the effects of suggestion. Homeopathy is thus relatively safe, although the need for a proper diagnosis must always be kept in mind.

In treating chronic disease, prescribers set great store by factors that make the pain better or worse (movement, warmth, and so on). They are also likely to be interested in the emotional accompaniments of the back pain: tearfulness, anxiety, irritability, for example. Sometimes the medicines are given in a single dose, but they may be taken daily for a period of time.

Effectiveness This is difficult to evaluate. Many patients derive benefit from homeopathy. Critics argue that this is due to the placebo effect and other factors unconnected with homeopathy such as mistaken diagnosis or spontaneous improvement, but this is irrelevant for anyone who finds it helpful. There is therefore no reason why someone suffering from chronic back pain that is not caused by any serious disease should not give homeopathy a try.

Homeopathy probably has less application for back pain sufferers than the various forms of physical treatment such as manipulation and acupuncture, but this is a generalization and there are always exceptions. For people who like homeopathy and respond well to it, it might be the best complementary treatment to choose.

Meditation, relaxation, and self-hypnosis

As we saw when considering the multidisciplinary approach in "Treating Chronic Back Pain" (pp. 102–105), techniques such as meditation are sometimes used even in a

A SIMPLE MEDITATION TECHNIQUE

Anyone can try this simple meditation technique, and it takes only a few minutes each day.

1 Sit in a comfortable but upright chair, keeping your back and neck as straight as possible but without straining. Your eyes can be open or closed; your legs should be uncrossed with your feet on the floor and your hands should rest on your thighs or be lightly clasped in your lap.

2 Spend a few minutes progressively relaxing your muscles. Start at the top with your face and neck and work your way down through your chest, stomach, legs, and feet. You will probably become aware of sensations of tension as you do this; they are usually most obvious in your face, jaw muscles, and shoulder muscles.

3 Let go of this tension, simply by being aware of it rather than by trying too hard to push it away. One could think of the tension as a message that the body is giving about its present state, and the idea of the meditation is to register it – to listen to what the body is saying.

4 After a few minutes you will probably find that your attention has wandered – perhaps onto some worry that you have. Check your muscles again; have they tensed up again? If so, just let the tension go as you did before. Or perhaps you find that you are thinking of some quite neutral matter and your muscles are still relaxed. At this point you can stop meditating if you wish, or you can go on a bit longer by transferring your attention to some meditation object.

conventional setting. They may reduce stress and encourage mental and physical relaxation. Psychosocial factors, such as stress and depression, may inhibit the recovery of chronic back pain sufferers, so it makes sense to tackle these using meditation and other relaxation methods. There do not seem to be clear-cut differences between meditation, relaxation, self-hypnosis, and similar mental techniques and it is probably best to take them together as a form of treatment.

Transcendental Meditation There are many varieties of meditation and their origins often date back thousands of years. Most have been linked to religious and spiritual traditions, many of which are Eastern in origin. Transcendental Meditation is one of the best known of these. It was popularized in the West in the 1960s by an Indian monk, Maharishi Mahesh Yogi, and many thousands of people still use it, in some cases without any reference to its roots in Indian religion. Many other forms of meditation, derived from Buddhism and other sources, are also available.

Relaxation Some people have taken meditation right outside a religious context. Herbert Benson, a cardiologist at Harvard Medical School, became interested in Transcendental Meditation in the 1970s and went on to develop his own method, which he described in a book he called *The Relaxation Response*.

Research studies have shown that techniques of this kind can reduce heart rate, blood pressure, and oxygen consumption, and increase the electrical resistance of the skin (a measure of relaxation).

These are interpreted as evidence of the "relaxation response." This is the opposite of the "fight and flight" reaction in which, when we are confronted with an emergency we react by speeding up our heart rate, raising our blood pressure, and increasing our oxygen consumption in order to cope with the danger. In the relaxation response these trends are reversed. When carried out repeatedly, meditation is thought to produce lasting alterations in personality, behavior, and attitudes that make it easier to withstand stress. This is likely to help some kinds of back pain, particularly those that are related to chronic depression and anxiety. A lot of sufferers, especially women, have noticeably hard and tense shoulder muscles that are tender when pressed; they often find meditation beneficial.

Breathing and word repetition The commonly used Buddhist object of meditation is the breath. You do not have to do anything special with it; just feel the flow of air as it passes in and out of your nostrils. This is hardly a "technique" but more a matter of allowing what is happening to come into your awareness.

An alternative method favored by Herbert Benson is to repeat some word or phrase. You should choose your own; it might have a religious connotation or it could be something secular such as "peace," or even a neutral word such as "one."

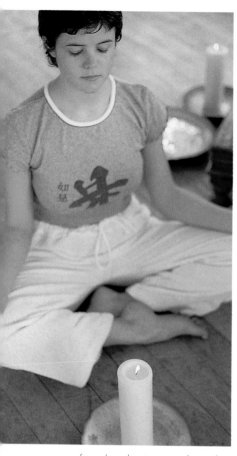

Meditation is unlikely to be the first thing that springs to mind when seeking relief from back pain. However, it can reduce stress and this can help to relieve pain indirectly, particularly if your symptoms include neck tension, for example.

But Benson insists that this is simply one method among many, and you should choose whichever suits you best. He suggests that you meditate once or twice a day; good times to do so are before breakfast and before dinner.

Whether you use your breath, a word, or phrase you should not feel distressed if you become distracted. This does not mean you have "failed"; in fact, it is what is expected to happen. Benson suggests you should just think "Oh well" and return gently to your practice.

Meditate every day As you establish this simple routine of daily meditation you will probably find that you become aware of the tensing of your muscles, even outside the formal meditation periods; and now you can let go of it immediately and the cycles of tension and pain are no longer so intense. The same meditation technique can help insomniacs who will probably find that it works best if they meditate lying on their backs.

In the beginning meditation periods should be quite short; perhaps just 5 to 10 minutes. After some weeks you may extend the time gradually, but do not force the pace. Don't think in terms of success or failure, and do not worry whether or not you are "going deep." Just accept whatever happens. Some meditations may go well and others will be difficult, but this does not matter. Regularity is important; you should try to meditate every day even if it is only for a short time.

Done in this way, meditation should be safe for most people, but be careful if you have a history of severe mental illness such as depression or schizophrenia; if you do you should not meditate without supervision by an experienced teacher. Even if you do not have such a history you should not prolong your meditation time beyond 20 or 30 minutes unsupervised, because you may experience strong mental, emotional, or physical effects that may be difficult to cope with.

Autogenic training

Autogenic training was developed early in the 20th century by a German psychologist and neurologist, Johannes Schultz. It is similar to self-hypnosis and also has affinities with mental yoga. Tapes and other teach-yourself materials are available, but it works best when it is taught by a qualified instructor, especially since it releases quite strong emotions in some people.

It is usually taught in groups. You learn a series of simple-sounding procedures, which are really self-suggestions; each session lasts for an hour or perhaps longer and a basic course comprises eight sessions.

Initially you focus on sensations of heaviness in your arms and legs, next on sensations of warmth in your arms and legs. Then you do the same for your heart region; you focus on breathing, on sensations of warmth in your abdomen, and finally on sensations of coolness in your forehead.

You practice the techniques at home between sessions and keep a diary to record what you feel while doing them. You are also taught simple things that you can do if you feel yourself coming under stress at home or at work. All this is quite demanding in terms of time and effort and you should not embark on the course unless you are willing to work at it seriously. Three months after the initial course you are asked to return for a review to make sure that you are progressing satisfactorily. There are also more advanced methods that you can explore.

Teachers of autogenic training, who are mostly health professionals of one kind or another, undergo rigorous training and will carry out an assessment of your state of health before starting you on the program. As with other forms of meditation, relaxation, and self-hypnosis (see pp. 131–135), the main value of autogenic training for people suffering from back pain is where stress is a key aggravating factor to their symptoms.

conclusion

Back symptoms, and especially back pain, are common, and many of us can expect to suffer in this way at some time in our lives. There is nothing surprising in this, for the spine is literally and metaphorically at the center of our existence.

Some back problems are due to relatively straightforward "mechanical" disorders, though even these may be difficult to diagnose owing to the complex anatomy of the spine; others, however, have deep roots in our psychology, emotions, and lifestyle. This means there are many different approaches to treatment and prevention.

At the most basic level you should have an understanding of how your back is constructed and how it works, as described in the chapter on structure. Next, you should consider whether your lifestyle is a healthy one in general: all the advice that is currently given to prevent diseases of the heart and lungs and cancer is also relevant to the back. Thus, stopping or avoiding smoking, eating a balanced diet with plenty of fresh fruit and vegetables, taking an adequate amount of exercise regularly, and keeping your weight within the guidelines for your height will all tend to reduce the chances that you will suffer from back problems. And even if you have no symptoms you should be aware of the best way to use your back. This becomes important as you age and "wear and tear" changes inevitably begin to accumulate in your spine.

Even if you take all these precautions, however, it is quite possible that you will have an episode of back pain at some time in your life. The chances are that you will recover from this within a fairly short time, but you will naturally want to know how to prevent a recurrence in the future. It would be sensible to take this episode as a warning to review your circumstances and lifestyle to see if you can correct anything that is wrong. Equally, however, you should also avoid thinking of yourself in any sense as an invalid. Many people have one or two attacks of back pain during their lives but function perfectly well the rest of the time.

You may find yourself to be one of the relatively small number of people who have repeated attacks of pain or even are in pain most of the time. If this is your case you will naturally think first of finding a cure, and certainly it makes sense to explore the possible causes with the help of a specialist. For many people in this category, however, no definite remediable cause may be found, and at this stage it is best to adopt a different strategy. Instead of searching continually for a mechanical problem in the spine, think rather in terms of what can be done to alter the way in which the central nervous system (brain and spinal cord) process pain. This is emphatically not a way of saying that the pain is "all in the mind," but rather of coming at the situation from a different angle. It is here that the "multidisciplinary" methods used at a number of centers for the management of chronic pain come into their own.

This way of approaching chronic back pain is one example of a number of new developments in treatment that have come into existence in recent years. Another is the increasing rapprochement between orthodox and alternative methods. Not long ago these were regarded as radically opposed to each other, and doctors were not allowed to refer their patients to osteopaths or similar "alternative" practitioners. Nowadays, these restrictions no longer exist and many doctors have themselves trained in the use of osteopathy, acupuncture, and homeopathy; this is a trend that seems certain to continue and indeed to accelerate. At the same time, the complementary treatments themselves are being increasingly regulated, so that patients can be sure that the therapists are properly trained and accountable. All this is to the good, and so is the demand that all kinds of treatment, orthodox and alternative, should provide evidence that they work.

It is one thing for research of this kind to be done; public access to the results is a different matter. This is where the Internet is making a huge difference. In earlier times research reports were available only in medical journals and were difficult to understand for people without a medical background. Now, thanks to the Internet, authoritative summaries of this material in comprehensible language is freely available. There are other valuable resources, such as the Cochrane Library, which can be relied on to be independent and well informed.

Finally, what it comes to is that each of us has a responsibility for our own health. This does not mean that we should not take advice from health professionals. You should discuss all the treatment possibilities with your doctor, but in the end the choice has to be your own. The information provided in this book will help you in making this choice.

glossary

Ankylosing spondylitis — an inflammatory disease that affects the spine and some other joints

Arachnoid mater — the middle of the three sheaths that enclose the brain and spinal cord

Arthritis — inflammation of a joint or joints

Autonomic nervous system — the part of the nervous system that controls the automatic functions of the body; it is divided into the sympathetic and parasympathetic systems

Cartilage — a whitish smooth tissue that covers the bearing surfaces of synovial joints; it is colloquially known as gristle

Cauda equina (Lit. horse's tail) — the sheaf of nerve roots that runs down the spinal cord from the bottom of the spinal cord

Central nervous system — the brain and spinal cord

Cervical — to do with the neck

Chronic — Long-lasting (disease)

Coccyx — the vestigial tail at the base of the spine, below the sacrum

Connective tissue — a network of fibers made of a substance called collagen and containing various types of cells, connective tissue is found throughout the body; it acts as support and "packing" and covers muscles, nerves, and other structures

Dura mater — the outermost sheath of the brain and spinal cord

Epidural — outside the dura mater (Greek epi: on, outside)

Facet joint — one of the small joints between the articular processes of the vertebrae (Latin facet: small face)

Fascia — a thin sheet of connective tissue

Fibrositis — strictly, this implies inflammation of fibrous tissue (connective tissue), however, the disorder is not really an inflammation but is characterized by numerous localized areas of tenderness in muscles

Fibrous tissue — a general term meaning the kind of tissue of which connective tissue consists. Scars are also made of fibrous tissue

Foramen (Latin: a hole) — in the spine, the intervertebral foramen is the gap between two adjacent vertebrae through which the nerve roots emerge

Idiopathic — of unknown cause (lit. self-caused)

Ilium — one of the two bones that form the sides of the pelvis (not to be confused with the ileum, which is part of the small intestine)

Inflammation — a complicated group of changes that occur in response to infection and other disease processes. At the microscopic level there are changes in the kinds of cells found in the tissues and the release of various chemicals; clinically it is characterized by heat, redness, and swelling

Kyphosis — a backward convex curvature of the spine; a degree of curvature is normal in the thoracic region but the term usually implies an abnormal amount

Ligament — a cord or band of fibrous tissue that connects two or more bones

Lordosis — a backward concavity of the spine; there is normally a lordosis in the cervical and lumbar regions but excessive lordosis represents a deformity

Lumbago — a popular term for back pain affecting the lumbar region

Lumbar — related to the lower back

Motion segment — a pair of vertebrae, with their associated disk and facet joints and also muscles and ligaments

Motor (nerve) — a nerve that supplies a muscle and causes it to contract

Neural arch — the ring of bone behind the body of the vertebra

Neuralgia — a vague term meaning simply "pain in a nerve." Many kinds of back pain, especially those that are caused by pressure on nerve roots, might be described by patients as neuralgia

Nucleus pulposus — the jellylike material at the center of an intervertebral disk

Osteoarthritis and osteoarthrosis — both terms refer to "wear and tear" degeneration of joints, characterized by deformity, swelling, loss of cartilage, and variable amounts of pain

Osteophyte — a spur of bone that forms in the spine at the margins of vertebrae as part of the wear and tear process

Osteoporosis — a disorder characterized by loss of calcium from the bones. It occurs to some extent in everyone as they get older but is particularly troublesome in women after menopause

Paget's disease of bone — a disease of unknown cause in which bones become thickened and distorted

Parasympathetic nervous system — one of the two divisions of the autonomic nervous system, concerned mainly with maintenance of the status quo

Pedicle — the portion of bone that joins the body of a vertebra to the rest of the neural arch

Periosteum — the membrane that covers the bones and helps to nourish them

Pia mater — the innermost layer of the three sheaths surrounding the brain and spinal cord

Process — a projecting piece of bone

Prolapse — the abnormal protrusion of some part of the body into an area where it should not be; in the spine, it refers to leakage of disk material to press on nerve roots and other structures

Referred pain — pain that is felt at some distance from the site of trouble

Reflex — an involuntary muscle twitch caused by a stimulus of some kind, such as a tap on a tendon or touching a hot object

Rheumatism — a vague term, sometimes loosely applied to rheumatoid arthritis, osteoarthritis, and other painful joint diseases

Rheumatoid arthritis — a disease characterized by inflammation of the joints and also changes in many other organs throughout the body

Sacroiliac (joint) — the joint between the sacrum and the ilium

Sacrum — the triangular bone at the bottom of the spine that forms the back of the pelvis

Sciatic nerve — the largest nerve in the body. It is formed by the union of several nerve roots in the lumbar and sacral regions

Sciatica — pain in the buttock and leg in the region supplied by the sciatic nerve; also, by extension, other pain referred to the leg from the back

Scoliosis — a deformity of the spine characterized by sideways bending; in practice, there is always a degree of spinal twisting as well

Sensory nerve — a nerve that brings sensations of touch, temperature, pain, and other sensations to the central nervous system

Shingles — also called herpes zoster: a disease caused by the chicken pox virus,which has lodged in the nerve roots in the spinal cord and which causes a rash and pain in the distribution of the affected nerve or nerves

Spasm — contraction of muscles that occurs involuntarily in order to prevent the underlying parts from injury

Spinal canal — the tube formed by the column of neural arches and vertebral bodies; it houses the spinal cord

Spinal cord — the projection of the brain that runs down the spinal cord as far as the lower border of the first lumbar vertebra. It contains both nerve fibers and nerve cells

Spondylosis — the wear and tear changes that occur in almost everyone's spine with age

Spondylolisthesis — the slipping forward of one vertebra on another

Sympathetic nervous system — one of the two divisions of the autonomic nervous system, concerned mainly with "fight and flight" reactions

Syndrome — a group of symptoms that tend to occur together (Greek: running together)

Synovial joint — the most common kind of joint in the body, characterized by a capsule made up of fibrous tissue lined with synovial membrane; the joint surfaces are covered with cartilage

Tendon — a cord or sheet of specialized fibrous tissue that attaches a muscle to bone

TENS — transcutaneous electrical nerve stimulation: a method of pain relief

Thoracic — pertaining to the chest (thorax)

Trigger point — a point, or rather zone, in muscle or other tissue that hurts when it is pressed and from which pain may be referred to other areas

Vertebra (pl. vertebrae) — one of the 24 bones that, together with the sacrum and coccyx, make up the spinal column

useful organizations

Acupuncture
American Association of Acupuncture
and Oriental Medicine
1424 16th Street NW, Suite 501
Washington DC 20036
www.aaaom.org

American Academy of Medical
Acupuncture
4929 Wiltshire Blvd., Suite 428
Los Angeles, CA 90010
Tel: (313) 937-5514
www.medicalacupuncture.org

Alexander Technique
The American Society for the
Alexander Technique
P.O. Box 60008
Florence, MA 01062
Tel: (800) 473-0620
www.alexandertech.org

The Complete Guide to the
Alexander Technique
www.alexandertechnique.com

Chiropractic
American Chiropractic Association
1701 Clarendon Blvd.
Arlington, VA 22209
Tel: (800) 986-4636
www.amerchiro.org

The Cochrane Back Group
Chantelle Garritty, The Institute for
Work and Health
481 University Avenue, Suite 800
Toronto, Ontario, Canada M5G 2E9
Tel: +1 416-927-2027
www.cochrane.iwh.on.ca

The Cochrane Collaboration
www.cochrane.org

Feldenkrais
Feldenkrais Guild of North America
3611 SW Hood Ave., Suite 100
Portland, OR 97201
Tel: (800) 775-2118
www.feldenkrais.com

Hellerwork
Hellerwork International
3435 M Street
Eureka, CA 95503
Tel: (800) 392-3900 or 707-441-4949
www.hellerwork.com

Herbal Medicine
American Herbalists Guild
1931 Gaddis Rd.
Canton, GA 30115
Tel: (770) 751-6021
www.americanherbalistsguild.com

American Holistic Medical
Association
6728 Old McLean Village Dr.
McLean, VA 22101
www.holisticmedicine.org

Information from the U.S. National
Library of Medicine and the National
Institutes of Health
www.nlm.nih.gov/medlineplus/herbal
medicine.html

Homeopathy
American Institute of Homeopathy
1585 Glencoe Dr.
Denver, CO 80220
Tel: (303) 370-9164
www.homeopathyusa.org

National Center for Homeopathy
801 North Fairfax St., Suite 306
Alexandria, VA 22314
Tel: (703) 548-7790
www.homeopathic.org

Massage

American Massage Therapy
Association
820 Davis St., Suite 100
Evanston, Il 60201-4444
Tel: (708) 864-0123
www.amtamassage.org

Association of Bodyworkers and
Massage Professionals
28677 Buffalow Park Rd.
Evergreen, CO 80439
www.abmp.com

National Guideline
Clearinghouse (USA)

A public resource for evidence-based
clinical practice guidelines
www.guideline.gov

Nutrition

Food and Nutrition Information
Centre
Agricultural Research Service, USDA,
National Agricultural Library, Room 105
10301 Baltimore Ave.
Beltsville, MD 20705-2351
Tel: (301) 504-5719
www.nal.usda.gov/fnic

Orthopedic Medicine

American Association of Orthopedic
Medicine
P.O. Box 4997
Buena Vista, CO 81211
Tel: (800) 992-2063
www.aaomed.org

Osteopathy

American Academy of Osteopathy
3500 DePauw Blvd., Suite 1080
Indianapolis, IN 46268-1390
Tel: (317) 879-0563
www.academyofosteopathy.org

Pain

American Pain Foundation
201 N. Charles St., Suite 710

Baltimore, MD 21201-4111
Tel: 1-888-615-PAIN (7246)
Email: info@painfoundation.org

Physiotherapy

American Physical Therapy
Association
1111 North Fairfax St.
Alexandria, VA 22314-1488
Tel: (703) 684-2782
www.apta.org

Pilates

The Pilates Studio
2121 Broadway, Suite 201
New York, NY 10023
Tel: (212) 875-0189
www.pilatesstudio.com
www.pilatesguild.com

Podiatry

American Podiatric Medical
Association
9312 Old Georgetown Rd.
Bethesda, MD 20814
Tel: (301) 571-9200
www.apma.org

Psychology

American Psychological Association
750 First St., NE
Washington, DC 20002
Tel: (415) 327-2066.
www.apa.org

Rolfing

The Rolf Institute
205 Canyon Blvd.
Boulder, CO 80302
Tel: (800) 530-8875
www.rolf.org

Yoga and Meditation

International Association of
Yoga Therapists
109 Hillside Ave.
Mill Valley, CA 94941
www.iayt.org

index